MELTZER IN VENICE

Working with Meltzer Series

Forthcoming:

Meltzer in São Paulo
edited by Marisa Melega

Meltzer in Paris
edited by Didier Houzel and Bianca Lechevalier

Already published by Karnac:

Psychoanalytic Work with Children and Adults: Meltzer in Barcelona
edited by Donald Meltzer

The Simsbury Seminars
edited by Rosa Castella, Lluis Farré, and Carlos Tabbia

MELTZER IN VENICE

SEMINARS WITH
THE RACKER GROUP OF VENICE

Edited by

Maria Elena Petrilli, Hugo Màrquez,
and Mauro Rossetti

published for

The Harris Meltzer Trust

by

KARNAC

Published for The Harris Meltzer Trust by
Karnac Books Ltd, 118 Finchley Road, London NW3 5HT

Series editor Meg Harris Williams

Case histories published in Italian in *Lavorando con Meltzer*
by Armando, Rome, 1998

British Library Cataloguing in Publication Data
A C.I.P. for this book is available from the British Library

 ISBN 978 1 78220 4664

Edited, designed and produced by The Bourne Studios
www.bournestudios.co.uk
Printed in Great Britain by TJ International Ltd, Padstow, Cornwall

www.harris-meltzer-trust.org.uk
www.karnacbooks.com

CONTENTS

Margherita Furlanetto is a professional educator; from 1990 she has been in charge of school projects for Venice Town Council which help adolescents and their families in difficulty, and from 1994 she has directed relational and school support groups for adolescents. She also plans, organises, and carries out prevention projects for schools.

Monica Longhi is a professional educator; from 1990 she has been in charge of school projects for Venice Town Council which help adolescents and their families in difficulty. Since 1990 she has also organised and conducted educational and relational groups for parents, provided consultation for individuals and couples, and participated in the implementation of local prevention projects.

Annamaria Mariuccia is a psychologist (BSc Padua) and psychotherapist, training at the International Institute for Analytical Social Psychology, Venice. She has had supervision from Donald Meltzer and Antonino Ferro. She lives and works at Bassano di Grappa as an independent psychologist, and as consultant and supervisor for various schools and community centres.

Hugo Màrquez is a psychologist and psychoanalytic psycho-therapist. He started his career in Rosario, Argentina, and after moving to Italy completed his psychotherapy training in Padua. In 1986, together with Mauro Rossetti and Maria Elena Petrilli, founded the Racker Study Group which organises seminars and training courses for psychologists and therapists working in social-psychological institutions in the Veneto region. He has worked with Meltzer since 1988 and together with Mauro Rossetti edited *Lavorando con Meltzer – Clinca del Claustrum* (1998). He lives and works in Venice as a psychotherapist and trains younger therapists.

Donald Meltzer (d. 2004) was a British psychoanalyst, origi-nally from New York, who taught widely in many countries in both Europe and America. He is the author of many influen-tial books, including *The Psychoanalytical Process* (1967), *Sexual States of Mind* (1973), *Explorations in Autism* (1975), *Dream Life* (1983), *The Apprehension of Beauty* (1988; with Meg Harris Williams), and *The Claustrum* (1992).

Giuliana Mozzon is a psychologist, psychotherapist of psycho-analytical training. She lives and works in Udine doing her main research with a clinical emphasis on child adoption. She trains individual therapists and supervises institutional services. She attended the activities of the Racker Group and Dr Meltzer's supervisions there for fifteen years.

Giuseppina Pavan is a psychologist and psychodynamic psycho-therapist. She lives in Pordenone and works there both privately and for public health institutions such as Family Consultation and Old People's Homes. She is a regular member of the training seminars of the Racker Group.

Maria Elena Petrilli is a clinical psychologist who graduated in psychology at Rosario, Argentina. She lives and works in Venice as a psychotherapist and consultant for Public Health Services. In 1986, together with Hugo Màrquez and Mauro

Rossetti, she founded the Racker Study Group, an association of psychotherapists from various fields of specialisation, in order to explore object relations theory in depth in the transference-countertransference. She has chaired numerous seminars with different authors, among which Dr Meltzer was a regular invited speaker for more than fifteen years.

Elena Pianezzola is a psychotherapist (BSc Padua), training at the International Institute for Analytical Social Psychology, Venice. She is a founding member of the Bassano Association of Psychologists which promotes various training approaches and applications. She lives and works at Bassano del Grappa in individual psychotherapy and couple relationships as well as adolescent and child therapy.

Rodolfo Picciulin is a psychologist and psychoanalytic psycho-therapist. He lives and works in Gorizia as a clinical therapist and trainer for health and social services. He is a former lecturer at the Institute of Social Analytical Psychology in Venice and a lecturer on the 'Psychology of the Life-cycle' at the training school in Trieste. From 1986 to 2002, as a member of the Racker Group, he attended the seminars and supervisions held by Dr Meltzer in Venice with particular emphasis on the clinical applications of object relations.

Monique Pistolato is an author, and an educator-animator, with training in the social psychology of groups. She has received various national and international awards for her short stories and many of her works have been adapted for the stage. Among her recent works are: *Un'altra stanza in laguna* (Another Room in the Lagoon) (Ibis, 2005); *Un tempo necessario* (Necessary Time), (La Meridiana, 2007); *Venezia: Guida alla città invisibile. Dieci itinerary insoliti e curiosi per calli e canali* (Venice: A Guide to the Invisible City. Ten Unusual and Wonderful Itineraries through Calli and Canals) (Ibis, 2012); *Cari libri. La lettura condivisa come laboratorio di umanità* (Cherished Books: Reading Shared as a Workshop of Humanity) (Paoline, 2014).

Mauro Rossetti (BSc Rosario, Argentina) did clinical training at Scuola Pichon, Buenos Aires, and is now a psychotherapist in Venice. In 1973 he became a consultant for the Regional Centre for Drug Addiction; he is a supervisor for the Street Educators Service of Venice and for family consultation in Verona. He is a co-founder of the Racker Study Group of Venice and regularly attended Dr Meltzer's seminars and supervisions. He organises study groups on object relations theory and is co-editor of various books on Dr Meltzer's clinical work, and editor of *Mito, mistica e filosofia nel pensiero di Bion* (Myth, Mystique and Philosophy in Bion's Thinking) (Cafoscarina Press, 2008).

The Racker Group of Venice

The Racker Study Group is inspired by and named after Heinrich Racker, a psychoanalyst who emigrated to Argentine in 1939. Racker began his psychoanalytic studies in Vienna in 1930, but was forced into exile by the Nazis and settled in Buenos Aires, Argentina, where he completed his analytical training with Marie Langer once the Argentine Psychoanalytic Association was formed in December 1942.

Racker was a man of immense culture, an art lover, especially a keen music connoisseur. He was also an excellent piano player and worked as a music tutor until his psychoanalytic practice was established. He wrote a number of essays on Freudian transference and resistance to psychoanalytical treatment in addition to works on psychoanalysis and its relation to culture, arts and anthropology. But his major contribution to psychoanalytical work was his writing on the dynamics of countertransference, a topic on which Paula Heimann also began to work, although neither analyst knew of the other's investigations.

When Racker presented his ideas on psychoanalysis to the APA in 1948, he met with resistance from many of his colleagues. The latter at first failed to grasp the deeply innovative nature of his studies which were to revolutionise the theory and the practice of psychoanalysis that was then current. Countertransference, as Racker saw it, is not so much an obstacle but an instrument for exploring a patient's inner world, a tool to gain access to its primary experiences and comprehend its resistance in analytic sessions. It enables the analyst to understand and employ for interpretation his emotional reactions (such as anger, affection, boredom, dismay) instead of repressing, denying, or confessing them to the patient. In his first paper on 'The countertransference neurosis' (1948) he described the analyst's influence on transference and its transformations during the analytical process, pointing out how both the healthy and the neurotic aspects of the analyst come into play in the relationship with the patient. In his subsequent studies he distinguished two types of countertransference – concordant and complementary – by pursuing the work of Helen Deutsch begun in 1929.

In 1960 Karl Menninger invited him to become Sloane Visiting Professor of the Menninger School of Psychiatry. The same year he was asked to substitute Hanna Segal, who had after Melanie Klein's death taken on a prominent role, at the twenty-second International Congress at Edinburgh. But he was unable to join either initiative owing to being diagnosed with an incurable illness and died in 1961, aged just 50.

The Racker Group of Venice

The Racker Group was originally formed in Argentina in response to our need to advance our professional training, which was then interrupted as we had to flee the country during the military dictatorship of the 1970s. 'You were forced to wean too prematurely', remarked Marie Langer on one of her visits to Venice - the Austrian psychoanalyst being herself an émigré who had ended up in Argentina as a result of another previous persecution. She advised us to contact Donald Meltzer to continue our education.

In those years, as Meltzer used to visit Italy to hold clinical seminars at Novara, Biella, and Bologna, we would also follow his travel plans to attend his talks. His ability to humanise clinical work and present a profound understanding of the patients engaged us from the start.

Our patients must have felt the influence of Meltzer's teaching. In addition to private therapeutic work, we were also interested in the work carried out in various institutions with patients we did not see directly but came to know about through our clinical supervisions and discussions at consultation centres for adults, families and children, including the Street Educators initiative set up by the City Council of Venice. We followed Meltzer's wider seminars in Italy and, after forming our own smaller group, proceeded under his guidance with the more complicated and intriguing cases we had to deal with.

At the first opportunity we asked him to come regularly every year to hold one or two clinical seminars for a larger public along with supervisions for a smaller study group. 'Like a pirate' he sized us up immediately; we were immensely interested in his wealth of knowledge. This is how the Venice Seminars began.

Donald Meltzer came to Venice for fifteen years and received the welcome of our group – an informal, non-institutional group sustained through its members' interest and work, something Meltzer especially enjoyed. His teaching was done through the clinical supervisions.

Throughout this long period there was always a seminar open to all – another condition Meltzer appreciated greatly: his teaching being neither intellectually hermetic nor elitist. This was then followed by the supervision work for a limited number of members where we'd discuss in detail the difficulties encountered in our work. One of the results of his teaching was the publication in Italy of three collections of case studies concerning different matters: claustrum situations, adolescents in therapy, and patients in public health institutions. Meltzer was greatly satisfied with these books, for which he wrote a preface. Later, we also published a fourth book (*Venice Seminars*) on transference, adolescence, and mental disorder.

When Meltzer could no longer travel, we used to visit him at Oxford and discuss our clinical material together with some of the members of the psychoanalytic group from Barcelona. He would listen with his eyes closed, concentrating intensely, and was surprisingly creative during each case study. He would work like a combatant to dig into the deep emotional significance of what we were asking him to help us understand. Penetrating the emotional significance of the transference moment and producing an imaginary conjecture was his way of describing the situations under discussion. This was never based on dictat! He would always leave ample space and opportunity to carry on after his clinical observations. Our catastrophic changes are always important. Meltzer's way of teaching through demonstrating, showing, always had such an impact that we would have to come together again 'after Meltzer' to exchange our personal impressions and opinions. Meltzer meetings continued to live on a long time both among the group members and within each of us.

Hugo Màrquez, Maria Elena Petrilli, and Mauro Rossetti

Working with adolescents

Maria Elena Petrilli

The majority of the supervised material presented in this book is about adolescents – by age or mental state. Only two cases, presented by a team of educators, relate to group situations, but the following introduction will consider them with special emphasis, as they have a wider relevance for adolescence as a general developmental condition.

This is the second time we have focused our attention on educational work: this has unique features and has found in Dr Meltzer a privileged interlocutor. The work in question, which was given the name 'Not only homework' (NOH), is a social service addressing primarily adolescents with problems who cannot ask directly for assistance but express their unease in various ways such as interrupting their compulsory education, or through loutish behaviour in public and sudden outbreaks of anger. In each case the educators have tried to devise different strategies to open up channels of dialogue with individual teenagers, and have shown their readiness to overcome their developmental difficulties. In these situations teenagers' potential capacity to explode should not be underestimated, since they may easily be seduced by criminal organisations on the lookout for new recruits for activities dangerous to themselves and their environment. The Racker Group, like others, wished to explore the clinical significance of their experiences with Dr Meltzer and to seek practical support and means for a better and deeper understanding in their work. In the case of the Street Educators, the material does not come from the usual therapeutic setting of a consulting room; nonetheless, it helps to unearth and rediscover psychoanalytical knowledge. On his side, Dr Meltzer seems to have encountered in this material a powerful stimulus to explain and further develop his thoughts in the area of prevention.

It goes without saying that prevention is one of Meltzer's key concerns. In *Studies in Extended Metapsychology* (1986), he writes: 'Should psychoanalysis contribute in any significant way to the evolution of our culture this must occur in the area of prevention, which implies the need for radical change in our methods of raising children and reconsidering our pedagogic tenets.' One of the cases presented by the educators here deals with this question directly and looks into the rigid aspects of our institutions which hamper learning. Although we were familiar from the outset with many of Meltzer's ideas we equally knew his readiness to review them in the light of new material with which he was presented. In fact, he did not hesitate to invest both immense mental openness in examining the cases and rigour in applying psychoanalytical thinking. His mental flexibility helped us explore new grounds, without disowning the fundamental concepts and techniques of psychoanalysis.

As Meltzer himself notes in the preface to *Adolescentes* (the seminars about adolescents that he held at Novara together with Martha Harris), published in Spain in 1998: 'Group relationships are in many ways obvious and central in teenagers' lives, and only gradually, at around 20, do intimate individual relations begin to put down roots, arouse interest, and enter their dream and fantasy life.' The supervisions conducted on the educators' work seem particularly appropriate for illustrating two central aspects of Meltzer's thinking, which he started to develop at Novara: a detailed description of pubertal groups with their primitive mentality, and his theoretical and technical suggestions regarding educational, therapeutic work undertaken with adolescents.

Personality structure in the early years of life, particularly during the latency period, appears extremely fragile, and may collapse when adolescence bursts in with puberty. This is why adolescents are likely to oscillate continually between unruly and quiet behaviour. The first evident marks of this new age are outward changes in the body, as the child acquires the sexual body of an adult. Simultaneously the teenagers' environment begins to change as well: new spaces of freedom begin to open up. A new community, a pubertal community begins to form, which is entirely different from the previous one made up of parents and hand-held children. Teenagers, in the course of their development, live most of their emotional experiences in this new community. Meltzer observes and describes in detail these groups and establishes the first difference between the early pubertal stage and the essentially adolescent one. Boys in the pubertal stage still stick to boys only and keep watch over other boy groups they compete with. This is why Meltzer denotes it as an essentially homosexual group. These groups are formed exclusively by boys or girls who often speak in terms of 'us' instead of 'I'. As well as rivalry with other boy groups, this is also the age when the need to compare themselves with the opposite sex surfaces.

The major purpose in forming such a group is to counter the adult world. At this age teenagers view adults as a power group that keep the world under their control. In their eyes the adult world is an organisation of an aristocratic nature whose principal aim is to safeguard their own power. This is why teenagers all too easily sway from the infantile illusion that their parents know everything to the idea that their parents are simply deceitful, inadequate, incapable of resolving even the simplest matters. They see the world as a political structure where adults wield power and force children into slavery. They, as adolescents, are a class wedged in between these two worlds and despise both for different reasons. Sexuality itself is seen from this perspective as the essential condition of authority and part of the massive control adults hold over money, home, and food.

Meltzer at this point underlines the extent to which teenagers seem to be preoccupied with sexuality while in actual fact their primary interest concerns the broader question of knowledge. They want to understand how sexuality functions precisely because they want to understand how the world functions: they want knowledge to counter their confusion. The moment they free themselves from their childhood submission to their parents, from adults who used to know everything, confusion bursts in. But the inherent thirst for knowledge shows itself in their effort to disentangle themselves from that confusion, and acknowledge it appropriately. In puberty, youngsters predominantly group themselves like a tribe, with little capacity to distinguish good from bad. This, however, does not rule out a course of evolution. Their actions are often of a sadistic or masochistic kind, but quite unlike cynical attacks on truth that only augment confusion by building defence strategies, as is the case with perversions.

The war between sexes continues in this process of upheaval but soon a 'traitor' emerges, someone who has become the boyfriend of a girl or has ventured to build a couple relationship in his own interest behind the back of the group. These young couples then form new groups, the foundation of the adolescent group. Moving from one group to another is crucial because on entering the heterosexual group developmental potentialities become available. Some big dangers have now been avoided other than those that may come from the adult world.

The homosexual group is by nature paranoid while the heterosexual group, because of its concern for the other, prefigures a depressive state. The initial pubertal groupings are extremely primitive. They are based on cross-identification, each group member taking on identity through projection into other members. They identify themselves via one another rather than with the group as a whole. Such an identification process occurs through a mechanism of a dissociative nature. Each single boy plays a role, with roles tending to change continuously – one day an individual being aggressive and the next entirely passive. These elementary groupings function by trying to avoid any sort of suffering. The group does not tolerate suffering and anyone who suffers is cast out of the group, which is why Meltzer terms it 'paranoid'. Only later, when the truly adolescent group is formed, do feelings of a depressive nature surface along with the initial signs of caring and preoccupation for others.

Meltzer regards the age of the pubertal group as the highest point in adolescent folly, while simultaneously viewing the passage through puberty to adolescence as indispensable. However primitive one group type may be, he distinguishes two important functions in pubertal groups. There is a new space where a person can feel free, and despite its limits this new space offers the possibility to experiment with new relationships. Adolescents here have not yet encountered a true object of identification but they have room, a space to live out the experience necessary to shape their own identity. As Meltzer sees it, it is essential to find such a space, a material one, in the world where adults have no admission. Serious incidents may certainly occur here but parents at all costs must try to keep away from it, as they must equally keep away from their children's room at home. An adolescent is continually on the move between various 'communities' – that of his own peers, his own childhood position within the family, and that of adults who fight for success and status. But the adolescent might also withdraw and isolate himself, which warns of significant omnipotent and megalomaniac aspects. This constant movement from one community to another enables an adolescent to find his personal grounding. Without such mobility, if fixed on a single spot alone, an adolescent risks not evolving at all. The foremost purpose of therapy is to help the adolescent retrieve this mobility.

We have mentioned these features of the psychoanalytical theory of adolescence developed by Meltzer and Harris because they sustained our practical work in the consulting room and helped us become aware of new phenomena. The educators of the Venice City Council were working with youngsters in full puberty, aged eleven to fourteen: all members of that particular group which, as noted, bears the characteristics of a tribe and still has to make its way towards civilisation. Here, however, the youngsters came from a troubled background, from families with problems ranging from drug addiction to criminal records and jail sentences. Some are citizens of a non-EU country and live like nomads. They are the children of broken, sidelined families without a role model to encourage their development. The boys are often bullies and tend to conform exclusively with the law of the fittest. Their fathers are literally absent from their existence (either in jail or in a drug-rehabilitation community) and the father figure is replaced by someone else, 'a copy' as Meltzer appropriately puts it, i.e. the mother's new partner who fails to act like a father at all. It is certainly true that they have not experienced latency fully but despite this, now that they have entered puberty they are also overwhelmed by the bodily changes and are strongly drawn towards their peer group.

The educators devise a space for them to meet regularly, two hours twice weekly, where they can play, get to know one another, vent their anger while feeling safe and protected. Here again we encounter the significance of 'a different space' guaranteed by adults where youngsters can experiment with new ways of relating with one another. The sole adults in this space are the educators, aged between 30 and 40. In this regard a highly innovative technical element needs to be noted as well. Meltzer always stressed that even in individual cases within a traditional psychotherapy setting it is adults who must guarantee the constant and secure presence of the therapist while youngsters must have the right to come and go as they please. Adolescents are unable to keep up with the characteristic structure of adult or child therapy. This is one additional reason why doing therapy with adolescents is particularly difficult. Yet someone must play the role of the adult who knows how to wait and can safeguard the challenge. Adolescents may leave but adults must know to hold on in case the youngster should come back. Such an approach, a major effort when transferred to a private therapy session, can become much more readily feasible in a situation such as the Street Educators thanks to the structure of a social service.

At the end of the project 'Tender your dreams in a tent', presented by Monique Pistolato, Meltzer suggests the group should meet at least once a year regularly to follow up their development, all the more so as they have gained a 'degree of intense intimacy' through their common experience. The idea, though, bounces against a difficulty often encountered in public institutions where initially elastic methods could turn into rigid obstacles. While the experience described in the presentation was drawing to an end, a new educator would be automatically appointed to take charge of the group the following year. This meant taking no account of the special relationship the previous educator had established with the youngsters. Here again the question regarding the value of such an experience does not consist only in creating a specific space for the youngsters.

Meltzer further suggests a way or a model the youngsters should seek to stimulate their growth. He notes that in the light of their personal experience the group with that particular educator will continue to constitute a reference point, a model for their growth: 'It shows a structure which I without hesitation would define as familial.' We certainly knew that personality features depend on the learning models in a family. Moreover, it has been made equally clear that these youngsters' families could hardly come up with an adequate education model. But the group made an authentic emotional experience which brought in its wake as an inevitable component a structuring element of introjective identification. The youngsters have no doubt learned certain skills; most importantly, they have learned something about the way of thinking put into effective use by their caring educator who functioned as the object-bearer of parental transference.

In place of a fragile web of relations typical of a group, Meltzer seems to aim at the construction of a family structure with its distinctive characteristic of a more or less stable organisation. His commentary made at a supervision in November 2000 may help clarify this point: 'What is being done through the psychoanalytical method is creating an "analytical family" with which a patient may identify and find himself, where he feels he belongs and may stand in the community as a representative of this family; this is the secret of self-respect, something that prevents a girl from turning into a prostitute and a boy from a drug addict.'

With the idea of family we have gone beyond the primitive structure of a tribe, although the group mentality may well continue encouraging non-mental functions. This is also why Meltzer asked to preserve the work ethos the group had already established, noting it would be 'too strenuous' for the new educator to replace the previous one. He underlined again the 'intense intimacy' gained through the experience. Intimate relationships, in Meltzer's definition, are those belonging to the area of emotional experience, the area that triggers 'the thinking process.' It was Bion whose psychoanalytic theory definitively established emotional experience as the initial step in thinking, which is why feelings constitute the central nucleus of significance of the human mind. This is 'learning from experience' with its mode of learning entirely different from those in which emotional conflicts do not take place. It was Meltzer who taught us to read Bion (in *The Kleinian Development*) and introduced us to the clinical significance of many of Bion's ideas. No wonder then that throughout his own commentary on our clinical material we could often follow his understanding of Bion's ideas.

After describing pubertal groups in the context of the psychoanalytical theory of adolescence, Meltzer would return on later occasions to illustrate the theme further. The pubertal group is certainly a much highlighted phenomenon in the present adolescent world with its rallying cry and excessive use of advanced technology. Besides providing us with precise and illuminating perspectives on primitive groups, Meltzer followed the psychoanalytical work recounted to him more like a keen 'hunter' than a 'gleaner' (to use his own words). As he put it in the supervision of a case in November 2000: 'Young adolescents belong to a sociable community, a herd, so it's quite hard to come across a sufficiently developed sense of individuality; perhaps they do not even wish to have one, they do not wish to be seen as individuals but would rather be perceived as a member of a herd which protects them.' The web of friendship, however weak or strong, seems an entirely haphazard one. There is little cohesion and if any, it is to be found only in a protected space where aggression should not turn lethal.

Meltzer's comprehension of young adolescents coming from disorganised families had particularly impressed us. In his view, these adolescents had nothing to share except the fact of coming from deeply degraded situations. They would check one another mutually. In this case, too, loyalty appeared in the foreground with a strong penchant for blind obedience. What they missed was a community of purpose, of interests to bind them together. What Meltzer was showing us, the supervisors of educators, was a crucial point. Very often we also had had to debate at length with the educators themselves when they resorted to the belief that all youngsters were the same and consequently all headed all in the same direction. This meant losing sight of the conflict of evolution, which implied that we had to find the patience to step in to recover it. Meltzer used to stress the false similarities, false appearances, and offered a different comprehension of the sort of relationship linking these with one another. We did know that basic assumptions may surface in a group unexpectedly but we hadn't considered them with due attention.

Meltzer's interest in group mentality was also reflected in his supervision of individual case studies. In Sarah's case, for instance, 'a girl turned old' with a brilliant job as a graphic designer and in her second year of personal therapy after a long time spent in a community centre, he observes: 'It's as if she were actually drawn to a group situation rather than to a situation enabling her to build her own personal ties. This group situation is one marked not so much by a genuine bond or relationship between herself and others but by a web of simple, loose acquaintances, not true authentic friendships: people she in one way or another imitates, takes after, as though she formed a part of the group, were a mere member of the group, and all experienced in a rather vague and nebulous manner. It's as if she found satisfaction in this web not as a web of relationships but of security. This is the sort of satisfaction that does not answer her need for inner security, rather it's a myth of security: all these people, so-called friends, who can live and eat together, go to bed and share certain services. It's almost like having a series of places at her disposal, of houses to gain access to, simply on the basis of belonging to this sort of web, of being a group member.'

It doesn't come as a surprise that such a young woman should still linger in a web of fragile relationships despite her remarkable professional success. Meltzer immediately turns his attention to explore the transference and the patient's feelings of exclusion as she shunned the Oedipus complex, regarding her parents as mere strangers, members of 'a web of middle aged people who live together for the sole sake of status, power and money.' In this light alone does her personality come fully into the open, with major emphasis on her feeling of exclusion from her family life. If those feelings come under scrutiny and are addressed with due care and understanding in therapy, she can continue to grow and face the core question, that is her Oedipal conflict. Furthermore, this proves that the theory of adolescence, as proposed by Harris and Meltzer with its roots in psychoanalytical understanding, starts with Freud, follows a line through Klein and Bion, and provides us today with an elastic model to understand emotions, even the unheeded ones, which occupy a central role in therapeutic work. The above case shows yet again that adolescence is a mental state of personality rather than a mere chronological fact.

Meltzer goes on to remark: 'I don't know if the internet plays a role here or not but today there's much talk about webs and links which, however, have nothing to do with true friendships, with love relationships or couples. Such links actually remind me of a military type organisation, founded mainly on concepts like obedience and allegiance, where one must be ready to kill for a friend without being killed by one. So it's a sort of aggregation, a primitive association, a system of values whose founding nucleus consists in allegiance, that is, doing something as a duty out of a sense of obedience.' He goes on to note 'the sort of morality which groups or teenager gangs rely on: a morality where one should learn not to get entrapped, embroiled, because primitive values lead to actions but do not help construct the thinking that enables a true belief in such actions.' Here again a description of these groups comes in clear and fitting terms, and is an important warning for adults, especially those working as educators, against the danger of being drawn into and getting involved in such actions.

The adolescent community seeks to gain control over the world and consequently over adults through information technology. It is the young people who are computer wizards, but all too often they abruptly sway from omnipotent control to feelings of panic when something fails to work according to their expectations. The aristocracy of the computer which has set up a new order, a new web of loose relations, could just as well end up endangering the family structure and render it unstable. Group creatures live in a different world from individuals and consequently experience such feelings differently. Meltzer makes the distinction as follows: 'Individual thinking operates on wholly different principles, that is, on the internalisation of parental objects of admiration, trust and dependence. With the help of these internal objects, thinking transforms emotional experiences into symbolic representations while borrowing forms from the outside world as containers to be filled with significance. Dreaming becomes the basis for the transformation of introspective processes into speech, while abstraction and generalisation help the thinking process develop. Emotional experiences, along with their deepest matrix (i.e. intimate relations with other individuals) alter an individual in such a way that the organisation of their personality can evolve. Such an evolution is the result of admiration for internal objects, and the essentially ethical aspirations which they stir into being.' Evolutionary conflict basically consists in the collision between primitive aspects and sophisticated or 'work' aspects. The small work group has thus become the place where work can be carried out based on individual thinking that implies accountable judgement and thought-out actions. Basic assumptions still lie in wait but the task can be rescued and finally support the urge towards evolution.

The story of 'Not only homework' presented in this collection indicates clearly the possible extent of such an intervention. Despite the high number of participants in this work group and the rather unusual space of their experience, Meltzer says he can imagine these young girls and form an idea of the unusual time–place dimension of their work. He describes the educators as 'the authentic custodians' of the borderline between inside and outside. The time–space dimension is regarded as 'internal space' by contrast with the outside world visible through the window, occupied by arrogant young boys wandering in the park. Meltzer, in addition, notes that the sort of community that begins to form in such a situation sounds like the experience of the Indian tribe as recounted on the previous occasion. However, in the latter group emotions were protected and only very slowly came to be distinguished from the external world. They too were a group of pubertal youngsters.

In the case of 'Not only homework' Meltzer stresses the idea of a 'not organised' work group. He is actually speaking of a different sort of cohesion: one which relies directly on the attention and the personal interest the educators offer in the course of this experience. This is also why he insists on the importance of flexible time and space, which ensures tolerance without automatically demanding anything in return such as obedience. In adolescent organisations founded on loyalty the predominant feature remains mutual control, with the lurking risk of falling through a loophole. The sole options then are either to be crushed under the rules or to be kicked out of the group. Tolerance signifies the possibility of a different type of cohesion. The young girls in this group have found a room to live in and express themselves. As Meltzer notes, it is a space without the usual rigidities of an institution. The least degree of organisation is what is needed for this experience to stay flexible. The second feature of this work group is that individual participants bring here their personal answers to the work they are asked to accomplish. The third is that they work in silence, without clamour, unlike other group situations. Meltzer indeed considers it essential that this vital space should stay out of the spotlight so that the group can concentrate on its own concerns and the passionate relations at the very heart of its members' mental life. Hence the necessity for a secluded and well-protected area accessible only to those who take part in this experience.

Working in a group does not automatically initiate a course that leads to personal growth. On the contrary, it may often result in building up a pressure which stimulates elements of primitive morality whose herd-like tendencies rise to the surface: yielding to the motto 'everyone is equal' instead of demanding from everyone equal commitment within their capacity to work towards a common end. With the youngsters in 'Not only homework' we can see an accurate description of the type of web in which young people move and operate, with their tricks and dishonesty, and of the way their educators operate as a sophisticated work group, who thanks to their intimate knowledge and commitment are capable of encouraging individual development.

Meltzer would often remind us that we do not have a notational system like that of music and that other non-lexical aspects of speech are important in conveying meaning: 'We are not saying it but showing it. This is precisely the strongpoint of the educators in this service: their capacity to show, the example they offer, the passion they invest in their work.' The Street Educators provide us with an example of the music, the passion we need to invest in clinical work with patients, and which is most clear in dealing with adolescents and adolescent aspects.

Meltzer seeks his personal notation by employing a precise and deeply evocative way of speaking. His attention, during supervisions, is focused on the description of emotions which come into play. This manner of expressing himself has made us discover aspects of emotionality which we had hitherto not noted, but which then turn into a new tool for use. As he used to quote from Shakespeare's A Midsummer Night's Dream: 'And as imagination bodies forth/ The forms of things unknown, the poet's pen/ Turns them to shapes and gives to airy nothing/ A local habitation and a name'. Similarly, we can also venture to say that he has helped us discover something altogether new that was there before our very eyes. In his often repeated remark, psychoanalytical work too is an art; and Meltzer, through his thinking, has sought to build 'a house for our emotions'.

Note

Dates given after the titles of each chapter are those of Meltzer's supervisions or talks.

CHAPTER ONE

'Tender your dreams in a tent': a workshop for 11–14 year olds
(1997)

Monique Pistolato

The protagonists

O nce upon a time there was a group of youngsters: to be precise there were ten of them, five girls and five boys, aged between eleven and fourteen. I know some of them as they have been coming to this workshop year after year while others have joined this experience for the first time.

Put together they form a picture of a microcosm made up of different cultures and habits. These youngsters live in the outskirts of a densely populated city, in council estates with problem families. Many of them have an extremely bad relation-ship with school, continuously failing entire school years and/or failing their school duties; but among them there are also those from a very common family and with high gifts. In most cases, however, their families are marked by deep social and relational unease (drug-addiction, prison sentences, social marginalisa-tion, non-European origins, nomadic existence and so on); this is why it is important for this service to establish a relationship of dialogue and exchange with their parents. This is a choice made towards helping the youngsters' growth while supporting the adults close to them.

I meet the youngsters after they have attended short animation games in class as part of their school activities. In response to the offer to meet in a place to play together, to build something, the youngsters, intrigued, come to the workshop 'Tender your dreams in a tent' singly or in couples. They might be drawn to the idea of a world of explorers clad in indigo blue, of secret codes, Indian tents, precious jewels and whatnot.

With some interest and some caution they are to set forth on an 'imaginary journey of the world' in 72 meetings lasting two hours each, every two weeks between 4.30–6.30 pm from September to June.

Everything is ready: the room is in order; the white and red checked curtains, like a saloon, hang on the windows; an old trunk full of objects, maps to decipher, and with plenty of feathers stands invitingly and mysteriously in a corner. The hour is about to strike for the first meeting. I am excited. This happens every year when a new experience is about to begin and I wonder: 'Who will answer my invitation? What will they be like? What will happen?'

The past and the present

Five minutes before the opening, Davide's deafening, lacerating cry reaches my ears from the street, he yells at me arrogantly: 'Monica, wake up, hurry up, get the milk ready, I'm coming!'

Davide shows up on time. This is his seventh year at the workshop; although he has had different leaders, he has managed to keep up a constant relationship with this place. This makes me note his capacity to remember on his own the opening date of activities, for his family is not there; his father apparently has drug-addiction problems, his mother is quite adrift, and they don't care about what their son does or goes through on his own.

His voice reminds me that he has now turned twelve, has failed a year at school, but still asks me for milk. And now all my discursive digressions, fantasies and ideas cherished throughout the summer vanish into thin air. I return to earth. In five minutes I'll have to meet the youngsters. The real ones. And they will bring me their disappointment and surprise (many are here for the second and some even third year) at finding in an orderly room a new theme, new friends, but will most of all have to bear that there will be no milk as a snack as they were used to last year.

I open the door and hear them rush up the stairs like horses pawing. I think it's in tune with the theme. They enter like a whirlwind. Some hurl themselves towards the cupboards, some look round in silence.

Berta asks: 'Where are we here?' She sounds lost even though this is her third year. I look at her. She is wearing black as always and her face looks inexpressive as usual. I notice she seems to be lost in her obesity. I recall the way she stays shut off in her problems. Berta is a daughter with two fathers and one mother, but she is lonely. Her birth father lives away in a community (I don't know if in a psychiatric one or one for drug addicts, but I imagine he is in prison), and the other – the acquired one – is not there because he never cares for her. Her mother, of a tired, neglected and unkempt appearance, is away at work all day long, and despite her efforts fails to be in her daughter's life.

In the meantime Davide keeps shouting at me again and again: 'Did you put the milk on the hob?' And adds with deliberate pride: 'This is Walter, a friend of mine, you absolutely must take him. I was talking to him the entire summer about you and the workshop. I stand guarantee for him!'

In the midst of absolute chaos I think I must bring up the title of the theme. It is the setting, the metaphor with which I invited them to participate in this experience that should help me. So from my animator suitcase I take out a peacock feather and once all are paying attention, I ask them to sit in a circle.

I begin with: 'Well ladies and gentlemen, welcome to the camp!'

'What camp?' asks Teresa unbelievingly, who in her third year is ever keen to display her role of critic.

'I mean the camp we will be setting up together', I answer her with determination.

'What about the milk?' insists Davide.

At this point I start to explain: 'The milk belonged to last year's "Star Station", while today we are beginning a new story. You need to know that explorers drink tea in the desert, a tasteful and regenerating drink. Explorers wander about prairies and come across Indians in camps …'.

This brief description of the theme catches their attention. They even seem a little seduced by it. Oh the power of stories and feathers! Seizing that moment of quiet I tell them the days, hours, duration of our experience, and repeat the theme of the year. I look at each one of them individually and feel that what and how I had imagined, foretasted and thought to myself 'between the Thousand and One Nights and the Apache Indians' has suddenly materialised here and now in this group. We have entered the world of fantasy, we have crossed the border of imagination, and are off!

'Yes, but when are we going to drink?' pleads Davide impatiently.

'We'll decide that together. The camp will meet in a circle at 5.30 pm every time. We'll have dry biscuits just like true travellers and each time your task is to take it in turns to bring them.' I speak reassuringly; but inwardly I doubt if he'll accept that it is a different year.

For the initial meetings I myself bring a short supply because I feel they may not be ready to bring them or share them with others. But it is my set goal. The idea is to entrust every one with a sort of affordable 'toll', the dry biscuits. I thought this out after working with groups of youngsters for years, for I intend to contradict their 'costs nothing' attitude which has often resulted in smashing things or anyhow in the idea that they are licenced to do as they please. That's why most activities have come to focus on gaining a sense of value and on the care due to the workshop but also to themselves and others, and trying to cap the 'everything free' assumption that is probably induced by the gratuity of the experience.

So one of the first creative tasks is to make a pantry. My role is to keep the keys and distribute the food equally. This then calms them down and reduces their initially famished response.

Challenges

The first two months are over-heated; every single day brings in a new provocation. Davide and Walter always come late, boasting wildly, banging the door, and never fail to speak bad words or curses. I discover that Walter, tall and heavily built, has received a warning at school after brutally hitting one of his mates. He has missed a year twice. His family is absent.

Maxim, who for years has been coming to the workshop on and off without actually quitting it, is always moving around, and blowing an awful raspberry at whatever activity is going on, to show off his high creative skills.

Teresa, with an air of sophistication and distance and ever unable to stop wondering whether she is beautiful and ugly, reacts to her friends' provocations without control, at times even throwing dangerous objects at them.

Linda, who looks thin and fragile yet highly attractive, is here for the first time. She is very good at school, is used to being the first and the best, and in the workshop reacts to every hitch with tears.

Berta, with a sullen face, looks on helplessly without moving a finger.

I spend more than 30 minutes ending their rows and soothing the upset. Even my loud warnings fail to change things, other than feeling Berta's and Maria's sharp gaze which seems to question: 'Who is stronger? Will you manage to handle this?'

After yet another row amongst the youngsters, an image occurs in my mind of a group of lions and antelopes chasing one another, which means actually playing. The former group, made up of some of the boys, try to assert themselves violently; the latter, the girls, appear to accept passively every provocation. Instinctively I want to forbid such behaviour but for the time being I feel I don't have the power to change it successfully.

Berta, without moving, shows no reaction, not even to the bitterest of jokes, and does not bother to defend her own things. I feel she is entirely defenceless and needs protection but this fills me with immense anger, too. She seems to personify that part of the group or of each one of them eager to be subjected to their own destiny, with no choice nor possibility of self-defence.

Theo utters abuse, talks big, and addresses a friend forcefully: 'If you don't budge I'll smash you to pieces!' Right after that he lashes out at a girl: 'If you don't give me one of your biscuits I'll spit in your glass!'

Despite his loud voice and forceful manners Theo is actually a thin, slender boy with big black eyes set in a wild blonde mane. He is a Roma. His nomadic life of months of roaming is interspersed with static periods in a house allocated by the City Council for his people. He has been wanting for years to join the opening sessions of the workshop, but this is the first year he has managed to come from the very first meeting. He does not go to school; as attending this workshop is very important for him, he not only comes sharply on time but also tries hard to observe the behaviour rules which enable him to stay with me and others.

Theo, Davide and Walter appear to be competing to find a way to become the leader, as though they were looking for ways not to disappear into nothing, and want my whole attention focused on them.

Davide, at the height of his offensive behaviour, seizes a hat I've brought for the games of prestige and challenges me: 'Look how I'm pulling it to pieces!' He feels he has won a victory over me and looks triumphantly at the group as he crushes the hat.

I certainly am angry and respond to him firmly: 'Remember you'll have to buy the same hat again and I will remind you of it at every single meeting! I have a good memory, so if you don't I won't make a contract with you ever again.'

A month later, with this remaining a small unfulfilled duty between the two of us, Davide comes with a new hat and, proud of buying it with his own savings, surrounds himself with his friends who witness the presentation. He says: 'Let's bury the hatchet.'

And I reply: 'OK, peace made – your hand.'

This is how we reach a temporary truce, while every day keeps bringing in a new provocation.

The tables of the law

Two hours of the workshop are simply chaotic. Periods of quiet are short and temporary. The youngsters refuse to participate in the games. So we spend most of the meeting in unbridled clamour. I refuse to play referee to their rows, which always conclude with the same winners and the same losers. They seem to want fights more than anything else: then we shall fight! But I allow none of them to hurt others, destroy or smash others' things, or run away from the workshop. These rules must be observed.

Then I focus on setting up arm-wrestling tournaments for the strong, speed tests to pick the quick and nimble, intelligence games to encourage the brainy, and finally, in order to steer and channel all that energy, start Indian hunting games with precision shooting. By offering each one a suitable play container I hope they will be able to express but also restrain their hidden, impulsive parts.

Many of those situations of apathy or over-excitement appear to lessen. Each participant can try to single out their 'strong' but also 'fragile' points in different camps. They begin to find out about themselves reciprocally. However, I notice that they are displaying their talents and weak spots to me in particular. And it is the game of transgression that they enjoy best and that proves most difficult for me to control.

It is Berta, looking like a massive tortoise, who in her role as the camp scribe, suggests from the place where she is always seated: 'Monica, your words aren't enough here! We need the tables of the law for the survival of the village!'

So I assemble the 'Indian Council' to go through every single rule of our initial contract in detail.

Every council member comes up with a good idea. They put themselves in the place of the village police and opt for restrictive measures and clear prohibitions. I'm put in a position where I have to negotiate between unlikely suggestions in a heated, tiring debate.

'Whoever hurts someone will be tied to the camp totem and tortured!'

'Whoever hurts someone will have to deal with me and may have their contract suspended!'

'Whoever forgets to bring the biscuits when it is their turn to do so will have no snacks for a whole month!'

'Whoever forgets to bring the biscuits will have to fix another date to bring them!'

'Boys who behave brutally will be thrown out!'

'Boys must try and behave more gently and girls, without being just as brutal, must bite back!'

I let them give voice to all their fantasies, knowing full well that all those rules will be forgotten in five minutes, but also try to find means to accommodate feasible norms. Once agreed upon, I will have to make them adhere to those group decisions.

This discussion changes something. Everyone is more aware of the others, perhaps for the sake of pointing out others' mistakes, but nonetheless more restrained, bearing in mind their collective pledge to the rules. Monica's rules are no longer in effect; what has now become an Indian camp is ruled by the group laws and by whoever, now more knowingly, has decided to play this game together with others. The tables of the law are then written out and hung on the wall. On closer inspection they do resemble the Tablets of Moses! I will need to work hard in order to get my wandering people to abide by them.

Donald Meltzer: Clearly we are going to see some stages of civilisation developing here. It starts out like people living in caves, hunting, killing one another, the men subduing the women and the women either loving or hating it but submitting to it. Then there is a call for order, and all of it is immediately put onto Monica: she is supposed to be the king or the queen and to rule. But to rule this unrulable horde is not possible. So the next step is for them to try to create the Ten Commandments, as Monica says, and the fat girl – Berta – is the Aaron to Monica's Moses. That's where we are at present. It has gone through these three stages very rapidly – I don't know how many days this has taken?

MP: Two months.

DM: Well the Jews took longer than that.

There is a move afoot, though it is not very clear, to transform the group into one of vigilantes, with everybody policing every-body else; it's an invitation to fascism. We don't know what will happen with that. It is very attractive; it appeals mainly to the boys, but also to the girls, who would like to rule as a group, and to impose commandments on these unruly boys. But they are still searching for a principle of organisation. They want organ-isation mainly to control the aggression. Of course most of them come from fairly disorganised family structures, in some way marginalised by the community – living in community facilities, council houses. The fathers in particular seem to be duplicated – two fathers, one of them away in jail or mental hospital or absent. So they don't have a background of family organisation to bring with them.

The metaphor that is being used as the materialist basis of this little civilisation is biscuits and feathers. I suppose these represent the food supply and the possibility of sexual display. Very close to the animal kingdom. The overriding metaphor is the Indian camp. Speaking as an American historian I think it is not at first sight likely to be a very successful one owing to the colonial suppression of Indians by the white man through brutality and deception, with the assumption of superiority not just of organisation and material possessions such as guns but also of intelligence.

Of course in relation to this actual group of children the meta-phor is fairly appropriate because there is clearly a distribution of intelligence, a distribution of the degree of self control, and of the level of civilisation in terms of capacity for communication. So Monica has a series of roles imposed on her: prince, prophet and so on, and the duty to prevent human sacrifice.

So far it seems to me there has been one event that has broken out of this metaphor of biscuits and feathers; and that is the episode of Davide and the hat. This is very similar to Moses coming down and finding the Jews had built a golden idol and were sacrificing to Moloch or some demon god and betraying the God of creation. It seems to me that that event possibly corresponds to the arising of art as an extension of the original metaphor of biscuits and feathers. Of course Davide didn't make the hat but he did select it, and probably selected it according to his own sensibility and aesthetic ideas. Was it Monica's hat he destroyed?

MP: No, just a play hat.

DM: Were there other hats as well?

MP: Yes, but it was a precious one, it cost a lot of money.

DM: It seems to me to be a striking departure from the civilisation that has been set up with biscuits and feathers; and involves the ideas of creativity and of conscience, and promotes the role of aesthetic appreciation. In a sense a new principle has been introduced here, of which Davide was very proud really. He selected the hat from an endless range of hats that were available on the market as it were. The conjuring trick is first cousin to aesthetic creativity. It's what Shakespeare calls taking airy nothings and giving them a local habitation and a name – that's the function of art, to make something out of nothing.

The place of the artist in a civilisation means that he is naturally the object of both intense admiration and intense hostility. The distinction between the artist and the conjuror is never very firm; it is felt that the artist is deceiving everybody – this is particularly the case with modern art, where people tend to feel the artist is performing a conjuring trick and offering things of no value as if they were precious.

We have reached a very precarious stage of civilisation where it is obvious that Monica is in favour of having some kind of rules, but these rules also play into the hands of a vigilante group of tough boys who like to impose the rules and take pleasure in catching the criminals red-handed. So it is very unstable and easily degenerates into fascism, and doesn't easily rigidify into a religion because it is very fluid. We will see what happens now. It is really quite exciting I must say.

Double identity

At this stage I'm being subjected to all sorts of trials to keep control; my own attempts to make them abide by their rules too often lead to even more elaborate provocations. I feel disheartened by the ineffectiveness of my warnings and I am about to resort to irony at my imminent failure; I can no longer hold my tongue when Davide spits once again: 'Now, we have to admit that an Indian piglet lives in this camp!'

Their laughter conceals a tiny dose of irony which opens up different ways of dealing with one another, which the group readily takes up as a new game. Maxim becomes 'the Indian skunk' because of blowing a raspberry. Walter, because of his late arrival and laziness, gets labelled 'the Indian yobbo.' And so forth.

The group then begins to generate more ambitious roles as well; for instance, 'the Indian skunk' then became 'the speedy Indian' and the 'Indian piglet' became an 'Indian inventor', etc. With their double 'Indian identity' every one seems to own their negative prowess but also aspires to a more positive image. This is how every Indian in the group starts to personify themselves through their double talents in the village.

Not everyone accepts this game, however. Theo's motto goes: 'He who hits hardest and best is the one who rules the world.' He does not respond to discussion or debate but only with his fist and more challenges. I also notice that the more he behaves as a bully to his friends, the further does he yield, on an imaginary level, with love and immense care to the products of the group. I watch him eagerly while his wondering gaze of someone who has never had the time and opportunity to play veers between that of a puppy and a bully.

The group, by contrast, respond impatiently and hastily to their own creative output. I say to myself: 'They cannot tolerate the time they need to create things. This is why they are disappointed by their own incapacity, which tends to lead to destruction. What shall be done?'

The most common words now are: 'More! Give me other stuff, I can't make anything properly with this. I shall throw it all away all, I can start again, buy it, it's the Council paying anyway.'

Now I wonder: 'But what is it they fail to make? What don't they like about themselves? What makes them lose their patience in waiting for something to shape itself? What do they want that's completely free of charge?'

DM: Let's talk about this 'double identity' and the business of assigning names.

It's not just that Monica decides not to expel people. It's that she has this device of assigning names to troublemakers, equivalent to putting somebody in the stocks: they were immobilised and everybody could see they were in disgrace, but that was better than capital punishment.

This civilisation has a certain advantage: that everybody is there voluntarily. They are like people who have migrated from the Third World to the First for a share in the riches, and therefore they're not really motivated to destroy the community. So we have a situation where there is plenty of crime committed by the less capable members of the group, but there is no revolutionary movement: no middle-class activist children wanting to destroy the whole system. The children here are almost all from a deprived population and this organisation provides them with an opportunity for play and supervised, non-lethal, aggressive behaviour with one another. They are probably not a very sexual group. The kind of sexuality that tends to promote the revolutionary movement has not arisen.

This business of name-giving as a civilising device is part of the creative impulse. In giving a name, a position is also assigned which can be modified: they can earn new names (Indian piglet becomes Indian inventor, etc). The name describes the individuals within the community and holds them up to praise or contempt according to their deserts.

The other function which has only been touched on is the business of mottos, of political statements, which are also subject to modification: 'He who hits hardest and best is the one who rules the world' turns into a puppyish attitude toward his products. You can see how political attitudes can be modified through the restatement of values.

You can see this social movement of the community from religion to politics is progressing in such a way that it will soon reach the impasse which is facing our present civilisation, which can't seem to find any value system for social participation better than democracy. The move towards slogans seems to come to a halt with economic materialism; unable to see their projects come through, they say 'Come on, give me some more material, I can throw it away, buy some more, after all it's the municipality that pays'. The big problem is for the municipality to collect its taxes, to support the community.

The conclusion is that there is no possibility of positive freedom: only a possibility of negative freedom.

What we're doing with this group is waiting to see what happens. Just as we have to do with our own efforts at self-government. Hoping that the capacity for thinking may gradually overtake and surpass the urge to action (whose most primitive form is warfare): that some sort of civilising of the community gradually takes place. We are now going to hear one of Monica's experiments.

The cure

So, assuming that each should take better care of things, I give a sweet potato to every camp dweller as a present and ask them to soak it in water so that we can have our Indian crop. This unfamiliar experiment pricks their curiosity and they show genuine interest. They prepare a container to grow their crop. At every meeting they observe the potatoes intently, add a drop of water; some talk about it and others swear loathingly as they see no visible result.

DM: On the one hand she is trying to teach them patience; on the other hand she is instituting land reform. Everybody will have a parcel of land, to civilise them – before they start stealing one another's parcels; some will neglect it, others will acquire it, soon there will be huge estates, and so on. Cuban communism.

MP: Slowly new potatoes begin to shoot, the slowest-growing tubers I've seen in my life; just when I was about to question my initiative of bringing live things with unforeseeable results, shooting roots and the first leaves surprise me much as Walter's unexpected remark: 'My new potato is born, now I'm no longer clean-shaven! My hair is growing, wow!'

The group is now apparently enjoying, with the new blossoms, a new pleasure: that waiting and caring can and do bring fruit. Perhaps they also have taken deeper root and have begun to change a little.

We now work at a certain pace, a little more time to build our Indian camp. The ritual tea-break with biscuits at the meetings helps to soothe bitter feelings and to make peace, once thought highly improbable. This is followed by new friendships. Seated round in a circle they begin telling one another their own school stories, their first crushes, problems with their parents; they are no longer indifferent, silent onlookers and begin establishing an inclusive bond with each other.

DM: The birth of sexuality – everybody has a sweet potato. They will all have hairs, the girls as well.

The roles

In the Indian game characters equally get more articulate. Berta, for instance, the sullen obese girl always dressed in black, becomes the witch; Theo, the nomad puppy ever eager for a fight, is the camp physician; the impulsive Davide who used to ask for milk and smash things turns into an angelic fishmonger; the shy Linda who used to cry for nothing and anything is now wholly taken with the art of jewellery-making.

Now I profit from such creative opportunities they've opened up, and try to get them pick the material to make the tent with, and get them to agree on ways and rights in order to obtain the necessary stuff to decorate it.

'I want the poles and the fabric for my shelter!' cries out Maxim, the skunk.

'I won't come again if you don't give me right away what I need!' goes Walter's threat, the clean-shaven potato grower.

'I'll give you whatever you need only when you are all through with your Indian stock: your headgear, the treasure box, ground sheets for games' I answer back.

So, impatiently but eagerly they start to get everything ready.

'The camp truly exists' exclaims Maxim with joy.

Characters of the Indian story each have their own physi-cal dwelling, too. Once the Indian homes come to life, they seem to put new energy into the profession of their own Indian character, close themselves in their cherished shelters, and work hard following a thread of that imaginary world.

Berta, the witch, makes a sophisticated truth machine and special amulets for all sorts of mishaps. Linda thinks out and manufactures a treasure of necklaces, bracelets and precious gems. Theo, the camp physician, draws up a detailed list of items he needs for his doctor's bag, left under my protection, and one after the other produces his white coat, overshoes, a thermometer and a stethoscope. Davide, enjoying the company of his friends, withdraws to his dwelling lost in dreams.

As more and more tents come to life with highly personal decorations and are jealously protected by their owner, just a few seem to lag behind. And I wonder how to get all the characters to relate with each other with the help of a new stimulus.

We then agree on a market date to invite the people of 'Cooker-land' (the workshop for 6 – 10 year olds that meets next door). They are to buy our products with the food they cook.

They respond with sheer excitement. So the market deal is commonly accepted!

DM: The potatoes were just a device to centre their attention on something. As soon as they have learned to centre their attention, their anti-social trends are modified into social trends. So the land reform didn't work as such, but it did give birth to local crafts. The next thing will be the tourist trade. Everything has its miscarriage – as Isaiah Berlin said, there is no one solution.

The market

Even the laziest and most stubborn in the group seem to like this idea and stir to work. Two months into the process of production, however, and as the great event gets closer, there are still very varied results.

The witch Berta's tent looks like a souk. Davide, the lazy fishmonger, has made only three fishes of salt paste after hard work; a whale with a wide mouth which, as he stresses while showing it, devours everything, and two tiny trouts. Linda, the jewel designer, boasts of a treasure trove. Indian Maxim has only a battered boat.

Doctor Theo's sophisticated bag, filled with all the necessary tools, attracts everyone's attention and longing. Theo, in his white coat and the stethoscope hanging from his neck, becomes an important figure. No one considers him a gypsy boy any longer; he is the acknowledged physician of the Indian camp, Doctor Theo. They all want him, want to play with him, adore his objects, and are thrilled by his role.

But Doctor Theo, once his bag is completely ready, begins to feel ill; the glands between his neck and ears are swollen. He asks me to examine them. I become his physician and as I realise he has a high temperature and is getting worse, he gets closer and sticks to me.

This suddenly overturned relationship seems to bode something else. I try to contact his family; after the first telephone call they 'leave the line dead' and to the second one respond 'yes, the asylum speaking' and cut it. I feel desolate and helpless.

In the mean time the big event is coming. I also try to get everyone to pack as little luggage as possible, without overtly intervening, so that whoever has produced little should not stand out. Indeed someone who has come up with little asks me to stand behind their counter. I do not refuse to lend a hand but also insist: 'You all have to care for and evaluate what you have.'

But I cannot help wondering: 'What are we putting on stage? Should I intervene? If so, how far? Will they manage to exchange their goods?' And I keep worrying about those who have a lot and those who don't.

DM: You should write a book about this. The fate of our civilisation is in your hands. Play is the clearest form of thinking really.

Participant: The hostility of the families is incredible.

DM: You have stolen their children. When they see the transformation of the children, it does make them feel that they have lost them.

The market exchange

And the market day has come. They stand with their open tents in a circle. The camp doctor is missing though. The tent with the Red Cross remains closed, to all the group's and my own regret.

For the time being I also get swept by the excitement of the market but hide my worries and anxiety for Theo. My only question is: 'Will they tolerate smaller children in their territory and their story?'

To my surprise, with their endlessly new and varied energy they act out their roles.

Maxim, with his paper boat, introduces himself as the guide of virtual tours. He asks them to get on board while making them notice the dolphins or terrible sharks. He sails through with his unique art: verbosity. Retail price: two biscuits.

Davide swaps one fish in exchange for three objects, offering each seller varied goods and multiplying the amount of his goods by three. The value of the whale and the two trouts is no doubt inestimable, which is why he swaps them with the art of an authentic merchant.

DM: Even the artist bows to the economic community and is run by the galleries.

MP: Berta, with her truth machine made of a box to put in your hand and receive a response from a mechanic arm, hands out short and pointed remarks to everyone. It seems to be now her moment to turn the tables, after being subjected to endless harassment, with the short notes written out for her friends. It is as if she were breaking the dark silence which shrouded her for six months as she distributes now to one, now to another, little notes:

'Dear Maxim, if you don't give up stealing you'll end up in trouble, so think while there is still time!'

'Dear Walter, if you don't go on a diet, goodbye to girls!'

'Dear Marco, now if you want to get on in this world, you must take out your …'

The attention with which these notes are prepared and how they come out of the magic machine seem certainly amazing, but they are all the more amazed by the truth of the short notes.

Moreover, they display genuine authority at play with smaller children in their chosen roles and are proud of their Indian camp. For the first time no one devours hastily the food collected through exchange, and all the booty is stowed away in the camp pantry. I can now see them as a group joining hands to do something.

Then I wonder: 'Doctor Theo, where are you?' Theo comes into the workshop just for me to examine his neck, forgetting his game, role and equipment. Until the moment when he announces he won't be coming any longer as his caravan will be leaving shortly.

A few others also simulate similar ailments in this period: sudden excuses, terrible stomach aches, bleeding and torn cuticles to assure a special dose of care-pampering. We do have an emergency kit at hand but no one is really hurt. They try to invent situations so as to come closer or perhaps to get more attention, and I think what they want is that special relationship they have noticed has been allotted to Theo. So I wonder: 'What else has this nomad boy left behind with us?'

Participant: Both 'Doctor Theo' and Dr Meltzer continue to exist and fascinate as doctors/witches. Even in Berta's case, for example (with her truth machine which dispenses those notes of pearls of wisdom, etc.) we recognize the role – increasingly getting more successful – of the shaman who can heal the ailments of a group.

DM: It didn't pay off in pleasure; the tourist trade wasn't brisk enough; the making of traditional arts and crafts didn't satisfy them. They are left really very dispirited.

Participant: But their talents have been recognised.

DM: There is this outbreak of hypochondria and accident-proneness, an increase in health-consciousness.

Participant: And Doctor Theo is not there.

DM: But his first aid kit is there. We are at a stage where the doctor as a person has disappeared and has been replaced by the drugstore, the pharmacy. A hundred years ago with the discovery of bacteriology and the arrival of immunisations, it was confidently assumed that medicine would cure everything. Now the doctors have just become servants of the government. There is Berta with her lie-detector; the witch-doctors will have a period of lionisation and be supposed to cure everything, but then that too will break up and a multiplicity of alternative therapies will come in.

The great sweet potato experiment in land reform and back-to-nature broke up into individuality and the tourist trade. Something is breaking down and becoming imponderable. The mysteries of nature, and the fear of these, gives rise to the growth of the witch-doctor and the psychoanalyst, with great expectations that they will save the world.

Now Dr Theo has been recaptured by his family, and he hastens to catch up with them and abandons the Indian camp. It is the start of a peeling-off. There is a collapse of *esprit de corps*. It will come to an end – the last one to go will be the witch. What has this nomadic boy left us with? The answer I think is: an impasse. The common market is collapsing.

Milk and coffee

MP: As the end of activities is drawing near, and for the first time, we set up two games in unison: a football match, needless to say with Indian footballers, and a pinball competition, again with Sioux decorations. At their inauguration, as befits the occasion, conflicts and competitions, filtered through the games, also open up. I imagine setting up tournaments could be a good idea for the end. Matches between single 'Indians', in couples, boys against girls and mixed ones can provide all with a chance to win and lose. The lions sometime play the antelopes, and the latter become the former not in a hunting game but in a real situation in which they get together exchanging different roles, and thereby also stir to life a part of themselves left dozing for long.

I ask them in the remaining months to help demobilise the camp. The demobilisation means a lot for me too. Next year I won't be leading a workshop. I will leave these youngsters but also my role as a leader to take up a new job. It is a painful separation; yet at the same time this gives me the opportunity to grow professionally and perhaps for them too to make headway in their growth. So I make the announcement a month ahead of the closure to allow them the necessary time to cope with the news. Oh! What an illusion to think that there could be enough time to leave one another! Once they express and shed all their anger and disappointment, they begin with questions: 'Where will you go? What will you do? Who will you be with? We won't forget you – and you, will you remember us?' The idea that after the summer, if they wish, they can return to a workshop led by another colleague somewhat encourages them, even if they all realise that inevitably it will be a wholly different experience.

So we dismantle the background decorations set up for a number of games, get the backpacks ready to take away for the summer months, clean and place neatly all the tools and equipment in peaceful collaboration.

Deep, strong feelings grip us all; for the work done they ask for a special snack.

So, at the meeting before the last one and assembled in our circle at 5.30 pm, thinking it a good and pleasing idea, I give them ice-cream.

Nothing could have been worse! But they still eat it ruefully while protesting about the tea and biscuits. I wonder: 'What's the matter? It's June 10th, sweltering hot – ice-cream is refreshing!' And I ask them: 'What would you like to have the last day?'

'Milk and coffee' cries out Maxim.

'Make it warm!' insists Davide.

'With biscuits' adds Anna.

I ask: 'Are you sure you don't want a warm chocolate?'

'No, we want milk and warm coffee' is the choral answer.

The motion passes with an absolute majority.

At the next meeting we say goodbye to one another as we sip with immense pleasure the sweet and familiar warm drink.

DM: What they have yet to discover through their sexuality is the possibility of family organisation. They will all want to marry you. And you'll have to propose 'Well we'll have to take turns!' It is very interesting and it seems to me you have handled it with great creativity. You have accomplished what you set out to do: these children have had a year of wonderful group therapy and have certainly developed.

Of course you have to decide whether there will solely be another group with another facilitator, or whether you personally are going to have an annual reunion to take stock of their development (which I would recommend). I suggest they have reached a stage of intimacy with you which would make it very difficult for another facilitator to take over – you will be a hard act to follow. An annual reunion would provide them with some cohesiveness in continuing their development – which has been astonishing when you consider what these children were like at the beginning, and the kind of unstructured family which most of them have. I think you have had one of the great experiences of professional life here. Now write the book!

CHAPTER TWO

Not only homework: street educators of Venice

(1997)

Margherita Furlanetto and Monica Longhi, in collaboration with Maria Elena Petrilli

In 1991 a specialist social service known as the 'Network of Street Educators' was established by Venice City Council, for the benefit of pre-adolescents and adolescents.[1] We established a relationship with these youngsters in order to help them with their homework, to help them plan a study method, make up for what they may have missed in their previous studies, assist them in their struggle to find a job after school, and support them through their problems. Soon we also began to invest time, energy and passion in an initiative called 'Not Only Homework'. This has turned into a social service in its own right, which takes place in two neighbourhoods in Mestre and one in Venice, and addresses a considerable number of children.

'Not Only Homework' (NOH) operates by creating a setting for a structured activity involving educators, volunteer workers, conscientious objectors (assigned to a civilian service as a substitute for military service) and schoolchildren. It also encourages

---

1   See also Chapter 1. Margherita Furlanetto and Monica Longhi are the educators in this chapter, written in collaboration with Maria Elena Petrilli.

contact with youngsters who do not take part in NOH but who simply look on, even if for various reasons they are initially unable to follow a fixed setting with time and date limits. We care for and dedicate part of our attention to the latter group of youngsters too.

Each intervention is highly individual, and a volunteer worker is assigned to each child. Besides organising and running the specific activity, educators establish contact with their schools, their families, and social services, if any are involved. NOH takes place two afternoons a week from 3 to 5 pm, and consists of two groups: 'the big ones' in their first year of secondary school and 'the little ones' in their last year at primary school. There is a fifteen-minute break when they play football, chat with us or the volunteers, try to annoy us by extending the break and so on, when they curse and at times smash things; others, though, stay on longer. Schoolteachers also volunteer in both groups; their main task consists in dealing with the homework assigned the following day, but also revising subjects and themes studied in class to make up for their weaknesses. They have an excellent relationship with the volunteer workers.

Up until now roughly 50 volunteer workers have joined this experience; most are university students, artists, retired teachers, and ordinary people, at times quite eccentric personalities – all, however, equipped with those gifts of patience, sensitivity, and willingness that are absolutely necessary to relate warmly to adolescents. As educators we are in charge of coordinating and running the whole activity; but we also follow and assist certain youngsters with particular attention.

Inside and outside

Our job is particularly relevant and precious for those youngsters who are partly 'inside' and partly 'outside' this overall structure. NOH groups meet in a ground floor room owned by the borough council with a big window overlooking the park; the youngsters who stay 'outside' often stand there and take a furtive look 'inside'. They are all well-known to Social Services, with broken and marginalised families living in rundown council estates; there are also those from a 'normal' family, where it is difficult to pinpoint a major cause or reason for trouble. These adolescents miss 30 school days out of every 60, barely accept the school structure and rules, and have difficulty establishing contact both with adults and their peers. They know some of those of the 'inside' group and are curious about what they are doing; but it is often our job as educators to take the first step.

In the school year of 1997–1998, in November, we noticed a small group hanging around outside the room overlooking the park. We would like to describe the story of our relationship with the children in this area, paying particular attention to Caroline (Cari to her friends), Jessica (Ica), Speranza (Eva), and Sonia.

Of the four girls we meet Cari first as she is the sister of a boy who attended NOH. Her mother asks us to keep her with us because she doesn't know how to help with her homework and that 'she doesn't listen to her'. Cari is in her first year at lower secondary school. She comes in herself, and then brings along her two other girl friends who stay outside the window and say 'This is a place for idiots! It's disgusting! What are you doing?' At first, we give them short replies; then they stop coming for a few days, or else come with their boy friends and kiss each other in front of the window, trying to make those 'inside' react to them; some say 'why not chase them away', some look on enviously, some get distracted and over-react. It is not an easy situation for us, who feel that adding a new rule at that moment would snap the fragile contact with the 'outside' children.

After a few days such provocations worsen and turn into genuine raids. There are now five of them: Speranza (not following too willingly), Jessica, Pietro, Matteo and Fabio. We feel like tightrope walkers for a while. I (Monica) try to control the corridors in the Community Centre, look after the caretakers who have been arrogantly insulted, and once or twice lead the boys into the room in order to get to know them. Their stories begin to emerge: Pietro, who missed a year twice in secondary school, is in his third year, still grieving over his father's recent untimely death, and with no intention of doing anything; Matteo's parents are divorced and he is dreaming of going to find his father who is now in prison abroad; Fabio, fresh from his third and last year at secondary school, is now working at a petrol station, but gets to work late and at times shirks it. Jessica, at first difficult to decipher, copies her boy friends; Carolina sits for a while with her head bent on the table, without a word, depressed.

After these encounters, I try to offer varied help: I'm willing to see the boys again to listen to them, if possible to help them fulfil their ideas (such as Matteo's journey to find his father), and I ask the girls to try and come to the NOH meetings. After these talks, Cari stops coming but a week later appears with two girl friends. From that day on they are an inseparable nucleus doing everything together, such as one day doing all Cari's homework, another Jessica's and so forth. As we feel they do not wish to be divided we accept it and do not interfere. Their school situation is as follows: Cari is in the first year of secondary school, Eva and Ica are repeating the first year. The boys however we meet in the park or in the neighbourhood; the tension has eased off now and having a chat is easier; in the summer they will join the various games initiatives in the neighbourhood; later on Matteo and Pietro will be assisted by an educator.

Individual educators now describe their experience of the children they have been working with. Firstly, Monica Longhi describes Carolina.

Carolina

Today she is nearly fourteen, the sixth daughter of a mother whom the court has appointed to adopt the first four children, all fathered by different men. She has managed to set up a family with her latest husband, Cari's father, including in it also her fifth son Marco (seventeen years old) who has serious incontinence problems (urine and faeces), who had always been in the care of Adolescent Psychiatry and a private psychologist until he had to be taken away from his home and placed in a community for juveniles, where he has continued to reside. Cari's mother is a big woman with a voice like a man's; she looks a mess and stinks of urine; her house is in terrible disorder, with mixed clean and dirty clothes all over the floor; an armchair caught my attention because she uses its ripped up pillow as a sort of utility space dumping in it cleaning liquids, polish, socks etc. Her father works as a hospital porter and looks like a normal person. Cari is intelligent, quick-witted, but her teachers criticise her for acting the 'primadonna' by interfering and criticising others. All too often she is upset, cannot sit still throughout lessons, and imitates a pregnant woman by stuffing things under her jumper.

It is late afternoon at NOH on a Monday in December, 1997. Cari finishes copying from a book and Ica tells me she has to describe people's pictures, so I ask Cari to help Ica. We sit down in this order: Cari, Jessica, Speranza and me. Everything seems to be going well, we are almost at the end and I suggest doing the final bit on Wednesday. It is 5.05 pm and when the girls look at their watches they are surprised by how swiftly all that time has passed. Usually by 4.45 pm they get restless, saying they have to catch the bus. Nearly two months after this we try to find a way to distinguish them individually: gradually and cautiously, we ask each one about their school day, their personal preferences, and try to introduce a work division.

On a Wednesday in February, they are again sitting at the same table. Cari and Eva have to study the Aosta Valley, and Ica is doing grammar; to avoid any distraction we ask two educators to help them: one for Cari and Eva, the other for Ica. To our surprise they accept this. Cari alone protests vaguely but to the educator working with Ica; the educator tries to reassure her, promising to be back with her in an hour. Cari and Ica (and less so Eva) try to catch the educators' gaze; as when Margherita says: 'They don't actually call me, but their eyes look for and ask for me.' This silent way of talking has only increased recently. They follow us with their eyes when we move away from their table, or when we talk with other children, and if we do not look back after a long while they get agitated and disturb others in the room.

For their geography homework I ask them to imagine a journey to the Aosta Valley. Eva shows the greatest interest and accepts the task eagerly. When I go back to them I tell the three girls of my own short trip to this place. They listen with interest and attention, and thanks to this opening I suggest reading the text so that we can make our detailed travel plan. I

notice that talking about one's own personal experience makes
a bigger impact on them and this is how we shall study at other
times as well.

Things go quite well for a few more months; we work with
them, and other youngsters with volunteer workers; we are about
20 in the room with the window overlooking the park.

On a Monday in February 1998, Ica comes in alone to tell me
that she has broken up with Eva. Ica's version is that because Eva
'went to bed with everyone' she herself did not wish to be given
such a bad name. Eva, however, next time tells me a different
story: that they broke up because Ica tried to walk off with her
boyfriend while she was ill at home. Eva misses the next three
sessions at NOH but Cari brings us the news that her father has
beem taken ill and she has to stay at home to help her mother.

Margherita Furlanetto now presents Speranza.

Speranza

Speranza is fourteen years old. She lives in the flat below Cari's
with her mother, Diodata, age 37 but looking 50 owing to her
shabby appearance, and her sister Fede, nine years old. Her father
is still in hospital, a cancer patient who has had one leg amputated.
She also has an older brother, Alberto (now seventeen) from her
mother's previous marriage; since age fourteen Alberto has been
going in and out of communities for juvenile criminals, as a result
of various thefts. The Court has ordered him to stay in a community until he is eighteen. What is striking in Speranza's house is the
cold and barren furniture: plastic flowers on the table, next to the
picture of her deceased parents and especially next to her mother's
father's picture. They also have two dogs and a cat. For some time
Speranza and her friends used to lock themselves in her room and
smoke while her father lay in an oxygen tent in the next room;
she responded to her mother's requests with a grunt. Her mother
is unable to look after the family; occasionally she cleans the stairs
of apartment blocks, often asking Speranza to act as substitute for
her. About ten days ago Speranza's father died.

I have talked with the social worker caring for her family;
the situation looks quite bleak. Speranza's father is seriously ill,

her brother has run away from a community and has at times run away from home. Together with the social worker we have thought of asking for help for the mother, a home assistant assigned to help her at precise hours of the day with the house chores and to help the children. I also talk with Speranza's mother to find out about the state of things and offer to accompany her to Speranza's school, for in one of her rare conversations Speranza has lately complained that her mother hardly ever goes to parent-teacher meetings. Her mother is extremely tired, worn out by her husband's illness and says in a tone of despair she has failed her children, she hasn't known how to look after them, and that 'we can take them away'. On our way to school she tells me, quite moved, how as a child she spent some time in an institution because in her family there were too many children and her mother didn't know how to cope with them. She also talks about her much loved father, who was mostly away from home as he was a lorry driver, and whose death left her in great pain. She also adds that Speranza missed several NOH meetings because she needed her help at home while her husband was in hospital, promising that she will come regularly from now on. This is how Speranza eventually came back to NOH and asked to be supervised by someone and to be left alone (that is, away from her girl friends with whom she has had arguments).

In the same month Jessica asks for permission to bring along a new girl friend. This, to us, looks like an attempt to set up the previous group of three again. We accept the newcomer and allow time to find a suitable way to cope with it. Meanwhile we get to know Sonia.

Sonia is presented by Monica Longhi.

Sonia

Sonia is in the third year of secondary school when we meet her, and in comparison with the other three is a perfect adolescent. She is beautiful, slender and keeps up with the fashion. Her mother tells me she has been a widow since Sonia was six and that her son, Piero, age 20, is now in prison for drug trafficking: 'a bolt from the blue' in her words, and she suspected nothing as her son had caused no trouble whatsoever. She tells me her story with genuine pain and worry which make me believe her. She talks little about Sonia; only that recently she has started eating little, that she is not doing too badly at school and she has never missed a school year. She gives the impression of a distraught person. I ask her if she feels the need for someone else's help at the moment but she replies that she is already seeing a psychologist. Piero is sending letters to his sister from prison, telling her to work hard and behave well. Sonia begins to tell me about her brother shortly before the final exams in June.

For some time we meet the girls all together and a little later some event brings Sonia into focus, and shows Jessica's desire to be like and outshine in their daring the boys who are a few years older than herself. One day a little before 3 pm, I watch two boys walk up to two other boys who come to NOH and ask them for the name of their friend who has allegedly stolen petrol from their motorbike. I know the boy they are looking for – one of the boys belonging to the 'outside' group and a friend of Jessica's and Sonia's. Straight after that two boys whom we don't know walk in and ask the thief's name. Jessica says 'I don't know him', and Sonia follows saying: 'I met him this morning and I think his name is Andrea.' As the boys grow more suspicious and keep asking more questions, Sonia replies with curses, uses bad language, and clearly shows she is defending her friend. Now the boys get angry and ask her to go with them to the police. She follows them provokingly and my colleague goes after her, with two boys from NOH in their wake.

At the police station, they just rant and rave. One of the boys says: 'Stop ruining a young boy'; Sonia, turning to one of the accusers who moans about no longer being able to use his motorbike, says 'I go everywhere on foot too.' Sonia leaves her personal details at the station. This ends the story. During the break, though, Jessica and Sonia tell me: 'You have done well not to disclose his name'; I reply I doesn't know the true story which is why I said nothing and that what worried me was Sonia's own attitude which could risk her getting into more trouble.

We have noticed that after Sonia joined the group, Jessica has found it more difficult to separate herself from them to get individual assistance. Sonia, in those two hours of work, stays with me or another volunteer, while Jessica edges up to her. Such intrusion at times gets more insistent. We begin to feel a sort of lopsidedness in their friendship as Sonia does not respond to Jessica's interest. It looks as if Sonia needs something else and sometimes lies about her excuses; in order to leave the work earlier she produces a note with her mother's falsified signature; but we tell her not to bother with such tricks and that she only needs to say she has to go away sooner when she wishes to do so. Meanwhile Speranza always keeps aloof and the trio relationship is becoming increasingly difficult to deal with. In order to protect Speranza and avoid any feeling of jealousy from the others, we decide to help Sonia with her diploma exams at secondary school. I also agree to meet Sonia on different days than the regular NOH ones.

This arrangement proves to bear some fruit. These days they often behave in such a way that the educators end up being against one another: for instance, the other day Cari and Jessica didn't want to come into the NOH room and told Margherita they were waiting for Monica; when the latter came, so did they. At times it's the other way round.

I begin seeing Sonia three hours a week, on two different days. Together we decide what to study and prepare for the third year finals. She is very interested in poetry; I remember some verses by Pascoli and Leopardi. So we get down to work, trying to understand the poets through games. She laughs when I tell her Leopardi was a hunchback and so ugly that no young woman fancied him. I occasionally ask her if she has had lunch, and she often says no but I do not press her to eat. After a few meetings she comes with crackers which she eats there, or other times a cup of chocolate from the vending machine. As we meet at 2.30 pm I also bring a sandwich and a drink and we eat together. So our exam preparations often turn into 'business lunches'.

Jessica shows us her school report card which now begins to have pass grades and even some 'good' marks; she sits at the same table with Carolina and during the break we hear them say few words to Speranza.

Margherita presents Jessica.

Jessica

Jessica is fourteen years old. Her family looks very much like the cartoon film the Addams family. Her mother has long raven-black hair, wears long dresses and keeps up the family tradition of reading cards; her grandmother and her aunt were fortune-tellers too. Her father wears his long hair tied in a tail, his thick eyebrows just like those of Morticia's husband; he plays the piano at a night bar. Her sister though is very different from her; she is tiny with short hair and piercings in her nose and ear; she has no charm, looks mannish, is nearly nineteen, has finished the third year at secondary school and to date has never worked. We form an idea of Jessica and her sister as two girls who have everything which doesn't help them to grow: they wear designer clothes, have had cell phones from the age of twelve, get 10,000 lire pocket money every day which goes up to 50,000 at week-ends. Their parents explain that as they themselves had nothing they did not want their daughters to have the same fate. We try to find out if they know about Jessica's school performance or if they've noticed any change of mood in her recently. They cut it short saying they have little time and that school after all is not so important as making money in life.

Jessica has told us this year repeatedly she wants to break with the family tradition of card-reading; she actually wants to become a social worker. Her thirteen-year-old cousin, put under their care by court ruling, also lives with Jessica's family.

At the end of the school year 1998 Carolina, Jessica, Speranza and Sonia pass their exams. We invite them to join the summer activities for NOH groups, but only Sonia shows up for a few days. From July to the following October I will be on maternity leave. At the beginning of the school year 1998–99, we contact the girls again: Speranza says she will come for only a few months; Jessica does come but stands by the window overlooking the park; and Cari seldom shows up. They also ask after Margherita, whether she has given birth, what name she has chosen for her baby. When we give them the expected news, they decide to visit her in small groups.

After a year of working well together, we believed, we preferred not to put pressure on the girls but to take it easy, although for Cari, family problems are weighing on her. We do not feel we have lost contact with them; indeed they wander around the room overlooking the park, we meet them in the neighbour-hood, stop to have a chat; I even go to Cari's house.

In the summer of 1999 I pay a visit to Cari's house and ask her to join the summer activities. She seems aloof; I then add that I have often thought about her and that I wish to know how she is doing with her family. After such words a certain dialogue seems to open up; she does come to few summer activities and in October she rejoins NOH with her old friends Speranza and Jessica. All three have just missed a school year. In the mean time Margherita is back at work and again with us at NOH.

Carolina and Jessica begin by wondering why we failed to call them all that time; we say we indeed tried several times but got no answer from them, but we are nevertheless happy to be with them again. They then ask why others from their circle of friends now come to NOH, and try to keep them at a distance. They continue: 'When did you meet them?', 'Who made them come here in the first place?' And blurt out comments such as 'that girl is an idiot', 'the other is an asshole', 'F. is retarded'. They then conclude they want us specifically to assist them.

We feel we are now getting hold of the thread which had been left dangling; and we bear in mind that they may have changed for the better (or the worse?).

Although I was away an entire school year I don't feel there was an interruption in the relationship with the girls; when we start again in October 1999, it is as if I had never left them.

This is what happens after the first few days: during the break Carolina and Jessica, with Speranza a little distance away, approach a young couple in the park; the couple don't seem to take any notice and Carolina begins pushing them. I walk over to intervene but they keep on pestering and laughing at the unfortunate couple. I can hardly restrain myself and ask them if they are having fun and they answer this is sheer fun to them. I say nothing more and the girls follow me to the NOH room as though nothing has happened.

Carolina now begins wearing make-up and fashionable clothes but at times still comes in tight baby-sized jumpers. She now has a boy friend ten years older than herself. Her ambivalence grows more visible; indeed she often undergoes a sudden change of mood; she curses, rages against someone, tries to frighten others but at the same time manages to concentrate better, wastes few opportunities and is fully aware of missing an entire school year because of her bad behaviour.

Jessica, apparently less mysterious and better at relating with us, is no less moody but we leave her to do as she pleases; when she does not want to do anything, well she does not do so and we talk. Jessica now observes us carefully: she notes with much assurance that those shoes do not match the trousers or that the lipstick colour does not go with the jumper. The strange thing is we do feel awkward, out of fashion when subjected to such remarks. Unlike us, her clothes are nice and fashionable, her long hair is dyed like a raven's and she always wears a sharp perfume: she is the trendsetter and her girl friends follow suit.

Both Jessica and Speranza feel sorry about missing a school year and wish to go to school with their homework done. They are now classmates so they can easily swap work, although it is Jessica who ends up helping her friend more than receiving help. Jessica also adds that at home she tried to study for an oral exam but failed to remember everything the following day. I suggest we should work out a suitable study method for the orals, which she willingly accepts. The two girls now enquire about high school too: Carolina and Speranza hope to train as hairdressers while Jessica wants to become a social worker. We try to talk more realistically, reminding them that they still have two years ahead and that Jessica needs to work hard to qualify as a social worker.

Speranza now lags behind her friends in her studies, has little self-esteem, and before trying something always goes: 'not me, I cannot do this'; it is as if any homework were far more difficult than expected. But when we do get down to work, she is often surprised by her own success. She wears her friends' old tracksuits, prefers black clothes and looks far less eye-catching than others; she is far more withdrawn and makes no attempt to look attractive.

From the very first day of NOH this year, Carolina, Jessica and Speranza walk right into the educators' room, take our seats, and nose around our notes and drawers. They ask about our work, what specifically we do and if we know this or that man. They try to 'mark their territory', also against other youngsters, as though the room were their own.

Monica now describes the situation when she announced the prospect of her own maternity leave.

Another maternity leave

Ten days ago, the day when I decide to break the news of my pregnancy to them, Speranza anticipates it; the moment she gets to NOH she says 'You are pregnant!' But I tell her to wait for the session to begin so I can talk to all three. I hear her ponder 'so it's true', 'perhaps she'll tell us later'. When I enter the NOH room, all three are seated and expecting to hear the 'news'. I take my seat and say I will work with them until January, when my maternity leave starts. I also reassure them that Margherita will keep working with them. After a short silence Jessica says: 'You'd better phone Margherita right away'. Speranza and Carolina, however, want to know if it's a boy or a girl and want to touch my belly. Jessica refuses to touch it and they all ask if I'll buy them 'Buffalo' shoes, a brand very fashionable at the time amongst teenagers. That day a very different and strange atmosphere envelops all: they stay close to me, keep still and quiet and we all finish research on the fall of the Berlin Wall, homework originally assigned to Speranza. When we finish I say I regret leaving them and Carolina answers 'so do we'.

There is now another problem to deal with: the social worker taking care of Speranza's family says she needs to put her under the care of a different family so that she can finish her studies and get on with her own choice in life. I think so too as I have noticed Speranza's mother is far too absorbed in her worries and expects her daughter only to mop up the apartment block stairs, something she has been doing since age nine. But I'm also undecided because Speranza is and wishes to remain close to the other two girls and her entire group of friends. Her group of friends are Carolina, Jessica and few others of her age from the 'outside' group, plus five or six young men aged 24 to 25. The three boy friends are also in the group. In the neighbourhood we occasionally see the girls standing before the boys' medium sized cars, fitted out with spoilers and exhaust mufflers. We know the details because they tell us about them, how they meet in the evenings and stay up until midnight, smoke pot, and go on trips in the mountains. We as educators worry about the trouble they may run into; but we also suspect that a different environment or a foster family could result in distancing Speranza from her life, her own culture and her own dreams and fantasies.

Discussion

Donald Meltzer:[2] All this material can be elaborated and configured in these girls' mind as a distinct image. We first need to refer to our own experience in puberty and adolescence as a period of transition. On one side are the parents who are apparently there just to give orders and basic instructions like 'Did you brush your teeth? Did you change? Do your homework!' On the other are adolescents whose primary concern is setting up a web of friends, doing their best to keep them bound together, trying hard to integrate one with the other, and assuming behaviour which is not only acceptable but will also evoke the admiration of their peers.

Participant: It is striking how easily the girls accept this method of working; everything on offer seems to go down well.

DM: Perhaps to find an answer to many looming questions we need to look into the role of our educators, their role as the guardians between outside and inside; we need to think about

---

2   Meltzer's comments in this chapter were translated from a transcript.

the window opening onto the park, separating within from without, and the relationship between those who stay outside and those who stay inside; when those outside do everything to humiliate, poke fun at and distract those inside. The street educators become the authentic guardians of this border line and carry out their task with absolute determination, not only defending the inside from the outside but also safeguarding the difference between the inside and the outside.

We can feel the energy, the engagement of our educators in relation to these three adolescent girls, whose picture contrasts with that of their boy friends who are all of age and seem bound to get caught up sooner or later in drugs, stealing, violence or even sexual aggression. At the root of all this lies the impact on these girls of an environment, of a surrounding culture which apparently aims to produce men devoted to vice; whereas the educators' function seems to strenuously defend and protect these girls so that they should not get swept away by this wave of violence represented not only by their boy friends as individuals, but also by their masculinity.

On the other hand we see all these girls are the children of more or less unstable couples, characterised by the presence of inadequate mothers and fathers to admire and love, and whose union at any rate does not encourage the formation of a strong and stable family nucleus.

The name given by the street educators, 'Not Only Homework', stresses that doing homework is an active time; and the need to understand that learning is not simply a passive process.

Participant: It suggests the hope that it won't end with homework but may go beyond that.

DM: The sense of opening out, going beyond a boundary, that is suggested by the name, seems even more relevant when we consider that one of the things these girls do not have is time and space to do something by themselves.

Participant: The girls like especially the idea of having a personal relationship with the educators and getting to talk about their experiences. This is the thing they appreciate most.

DM: Regarding the sort of relationship established between the educators and the teenagers, I was struck by the communication technique, including the visual technique, because just a glance or a look was enough to reassure them. Glances that control and draw attention also to themselves. The way the educators try to establish a relationship with the teenagers and, in time, to keep them under control, reminds me of taking a dog for a walk on a lead, conceding a sort of checked freedom.

The educators' work is no doubt very tiring precisely because of the sort of relationship established with the girls, which leaves them an ample margin for movement, allowing them to come and go as they wish from this space created through the effort of the educators' engagement, passion, and time invested in this project. So much so that when the girls do not show up, the educators stay there calmly waiting for them, not knowing what is actually happening during this absence, what the girls may be up to outside this space, yet always ready to welcome them and start over again. Without counting the fact that the pregnancy of one of the educators becomes real news!

I think it's interesting to reflect on how this space–time dimension, rendered so flexible, could be suited to a more formalised psychoanalytical setting. Probably a similar point between the two situations – the psychoanalytical setting and such flexible space-time dimension – consists in the fact that in both cases the educator or therapist cannot use a formal organisation as a disciplinary tool but must rely on a personal relationship. This space-time dimension must naturally be protected in its quality of inner space, in contrast with outer space represented by what is visible from the window: the park and the activities carried out there, of which little is known.

In this way the question of tolerance also rises, which judging from the relationship between the adolescents taking part in this initiative and their peers, is apparently of little concern. These relationships do not depend on true intimacy but rather on complicity and connivance: just think how they take turns indoing the homework first of one, then the other. So if on the one hand we see the tolerance of the educators being brought out by these groups of adolescents, on the other we see that the girls do not display real trust in their relationship, but are simply engaged in a more or less fragile web of friendship where there is a sort of mutual allegiance, faithfulness as well as mutual control. These adolescents do not appear to have set up a community of intent or interest; the impression is that theirs is an entirely random relationship. Even their physical description, other than their personalities, does not seem to suggest the type of elements that could justify formation as a group: they have nothing to share, except for the fact they all come from a terrible family background constituted of poverty and degradation. We could perhaps expect Cari, as she has superior intelligence, to turn into their leader; instead this superiority only leads to the other girls' envy, who in in front of their friend, further lose trust in themselves. What is missing in this group, this random grouping of girls, is therefore cohesion; but this cohesion is replaced by the sort of friendship and organisation the street educators offer them. We also note Monica's pregnancy comes as a big shock: never before has there been this sense of intimacy, affection in the group; up until that moment the only pole of aggregation was represented by the outside world, by their boyfriends or other boys respectively. So now – by contrast – this internal space is created where their relationship can operate like a relationship among sisters.

The kind of community that is gradually created in this inner space reminds me of another case we spoke about a while ago, regarding an initiative of the street educators who set up a sort of Indian tribe which in time turned into a small community with its own rules and operating instructions.[3] Now, in our case also, what is taking shape here is a community which distinguishes itself from the outside world and where its participants feel protected: a space–time dimension that is emotionally protected and watched in an absolutely informal and elastic manner thanks to the educators' effort and dedication. This is underlined from the very first lines of the case presentation where it says that when the network of Street Educators was set up 'we also began to invest time, energy and passion in an initiative called "Not Only Homework"' – and I wish to stress the word 'passion'.

---

3 See above, Chapter 1.

Participant: How do the teenagers come to this service? Do they come on their own?

Educator:[4] They reach us in different ways: on their own, through their friends, most often on the suggestion of their school or through our own contact with their mothers.

DM: It's a wonderfully flexible space where you cannot be sent away as in school, family, or through the intervention of some social service; it's a place that works nourished by passion alone; by the educators' passionate wait for the girls who come and go and who at the end seem to be more coming than going, because this place is like a magnet, which itself is the result of the passion animating it.

If I understand well at first there were four girls, at the end though there are only three – the fourth has got lost?

Educator: No, Sonia has finished secondary school and we helped her get onto a training course to become a hairdresser.

DM: How many educators are you?

Educator: Four.

DM: And what is the core nucleus of these teenagers?

Educator: There are ten to thirteen youngsters at secondary school.

DM: So you are looking after this small group of girls within this group?

Educator: Yes, that's right.

Participant: Do they come regularly to these meetings?

Educator: Yes, although these were not very regular as there was a year when they did not come; after that they began to come regularly, although at times not all three show up.

Participant: What happened during that year of total absence?

Educator: From time to time we met the girls and asked about them at their school; I mean we maintained a line of contact, though a very weak one, with Jessica and Carolina, while we followed Speranza with more attention as her situation was much worse.

Participant: Is there a coincidence between the pregnancy, therefore the absence of one of the educators for a year, and the

---

4   The identity of the educators is not recorded; all were present at the meetings.

girls' absence? This could have been experienced a little like a 'rite of passage' from childhood into adulthood.

DM: But what does maternity leave mean, what's its significance for these thirteen-year-olds? This is the thing we need to look into. What's the leave from in their eyes? From school? Because this official, rule-bound expression 'maternity leave' comes from an environment entirely different from their own where all relationships are informal.

I'd like to go back to the initial phrase – 'educators who invest time, work and passion' – since this passion is the key to everything; perhaps due to the fact that the educators themselves aren't far from the world of adolescence and pre-adolescence.

Participant: I'd like to go back to what Dr Meltzer said earlier about how the adolescents were grouped, that is, the educators succeeded in forming a genuine group where there was none, even though the girls may call themselves friends. This reminds me of something that happened in the Veneto – a rave party where a young boy died. What struck me and made me wonder as I read the story was that many kept dancing even after the boy's death. This was a birthday party for one of the boys, so it was supposed to be something personal. But the birthday was only an excuse because they had announced it on the net and people from Holland, England and Germany came, turning it into a group where there was little trace of anything personal.

DM: I don't know if this has anything to do with the internet but there's much talk about networks, webs and links – links which have nothing to do with true friendship, with loving relationships. Such links instead remind me of a sort of military organisation primarily based on concepts like obedience and loyalty, where one is ready to kill for a friend but not to get killed for a friend. So it's an association of a primitive order, a value system whose founding nucleus is allegiance: doing something as a duty, out of obedience.

A link, a web can be formed that construes complicity, even connivance; in the case of our group, for instance, the girls were proud of the fact that the educator did not reveal the name of the boy who had stolen petrol, so they were proud of her presumed complicity.

Participant: Perhaps the group is standing on its feet because it's between us and them, between authority on one side and anarchy on the other.

DM: But first there's this web of relationships founded on allegiance, blind trust in the mates, where the imperative is to do something for one's friend, with no regard as to whether that thing is just or unjust. The cohesion of the webs of friendship, even the virtual ones, is based on their own ethics: it is allegiance.

Participant: How are we to interpret the scene, almost a challenge, when the girls shut themselves in a room to smoke while the father of one of them is dying under an oxygen tent in the adjacent room?

DM: Had someone asked them the question they might have answered: 'It might have been too dangerous to do it elsewhere while dad was dying under an oxygen tent!' These are primitive kinds of morality, independent of the matter of whether they are right or wrong. As such they replace the faculties of thinking and judging.

Participant: I wonder about what these adolescents have gone through and what significance they may attribute to this experience: distancing themselves from rather primitive modes and establishing a relationship with you. What I find particularly interesting is the moment when you make up your mind to tell them your pregnancy: I believe this situation could have given them an opportunity to convey feelings, work on something unconscious, making it become a sort of a seal to this process of education.

DM: I think the work carried out by the educators is so free from any form of preconception it is also free from any morality; all the same it could create a space–time dimension whose flexibility allows adolescents, including those with problems and disorders, to find a place to live, express themselves, however occasionally, and remain attached to even through weak threads.

Another 'virtue' of the web is that of cooperation which, however, does not serve to educate. The fact that two men work together to lift a heavy beam, something they wouldn't be able to do singly, is an example of cooperation, collaboration. Well, when the girls do their homework together they behave like these workers who try to lift a heavy beam: it certainly is a way to collaborate, not to learn something, because they limit themselves to rendering the work of learning for others less heavy, which is not an educative process.

In my view an important feature to distinguish and emphasise is the nature of the type of morality which underlies groups, gangs of adolescents. It is a morality where one has to learn not to get entrapped or entangled, for it offers primitive values which result in carrying out actions but not in developing the thinking that would make them believe in these actions. The problem with fascism, for instance, is not so much that it is a corrupt system but rather it is premised on the virtue of obedience. We mustn't forget obedience is also one of the Church precepts.

I am truly full of admiration for the creation of such a flexible space where one can come and go at will. I think you must have intuitively realised certain rigidities could occur and unconsciously eliminated them. I wonder how the same flexibility could be transferred to the psychoanalytical setting! For instance, one of the major factors of rigidity in psychoanalysis concerns money; moreover, when a patient comes just a minute too late, he feels he must apologise: it's terrible! It is truly astonishing that these educators have been able to create this free, flexible space without any rigidity: no cut-off, no either/or, typical of the norms and rules of institutions such as schools or social services.

Educator: Yes, but it is not always so; for instance, we also set time limits.

DM: Yes, but I don't see that as a cut-off: whoever does not obey does not end up in prison, does not get kicked out. Basically what I see is that you succeeded in getting rid of prohibitions, which constitute the pillar of educating methods.

Educator: Not always. Let me give you an example: the other day one of the NOH adolescents returned from the break far too late, at a quarter to five, only fifteen minutes before the end.

The volunteer worker assisting him kept waiting, we were all very worried. I certainly lost control a little but I told him: 'You cannot join us just for the last fifteen minutes!' In short, letting it pass wasn't the right thing and I added: 'Now go home!', because he shouldn't have been allowed to show no respect to the people waiting for him, to us workers and himself, as he wasn't done with his work yet. I explained all this and I sent him away but made my point clear; this might have been a mistake but ...

DM: But if he had refused to go away what would you have done?

Educator: I'd have let him stay.

DM: My impression is that chaos is always round the corner and that law and order are just there to fend off chaos.

Participant: I'm a volunteer worker in this group. I'd like to add that after Margherita's 'reprimand' – if I may call it that – the boy made up for everything, that is he was not left out. I also believe this shows the significance of cooperation between educators and volunteers, for we stood behind Margherita's message: that failing to respect a rule is something negative, and also let him give vent to his anger (I can't repeat his words now!), and then we asked him if he really wanted to finish his work. After just ten minutes he calmed down and returned with the promise he'd never repeat such behaviour and he'd finish his homework.

DM: Yes, even though in the expression 'work group' there's always the hidden danger of 'group pressure' which is applied through the acceptance of concepts like order and punishment. Work group work may also, in my view, be attributed to primitive morals, because it is also founded on loyalty principle, those virtues which enable the group to work as a team.

Participant: I'd like to note that Dr Meltzer is here pointing to the difference between team work and group work.

DM: This brings us to a very important notion of Bion: that is, the fundamental difference between 'basic assumptions' and 'work group'. The major characteristic of the work group is that it must be 'not organised'. The second feature is that the participants bring to it individual answers and reactions regarding the work they have been called to carry out. The third is it operates silently, without clamour, without showing off, without parade or propaganda.

Participant: This way of operating away from the limelight, today we could say 'away from the camera', brings with it certain problems; because this is a social service, however we may not enjoy doing this, we still need to 'sell' a certain way of operating. There are a lot of highly skilled salespeople who get on with simple catch words, such as 'obedience', raising a lot of dust and occupying the centre stage in social services. So instead of the term 'obedience', what keyword or catchword should we be using?

DM: The fact that something is for sale does not mean you shouldn't be selling it. The only good salespeople of psychoanalysis are those who have experienced its beneficial effects on themselves. A psychoanalyst may worry that too many of his patients keep silent and don't shout from the rooftops how much they have improved thanks to the therapy. They may not declaim it, fair enough, but they do show it! This is the type of marketing that you should rely on. Telling lies makes little sense – as we all know they get you nowhere, so their success is short-lived. 'New at 25% discount!' I'm thinking of the magazines on aeroplanes that lure people to invest in so-called tax havens: 'Come and become legal swindlers!'

Participant: I'd like to know how this model described so far can cope with outside interferences and not only those from adolescent groups. Let's say, for instance, if the social worker issues an order asking one or more of these adolescents to be put in the care of a community; now this would be interfering with the work, a destructive factor undermining the internal coherence of the group, regardless of whether one agrees or not with such a decision.

DM: In America the saying goes: 'Nothing can be done against community services.' As a matter of fact there's no need to fight against them: someone who seeks to look after things which are actually other people's business could also be performing his task adequately. The work group is not a revolutionary group, yet it is adept at revolution, though not as a group: as a group its primary task is being adept at work. A famous English poet used to say that great poets are the best unacknowledged legislators of the world precisely because the use of language, itself revolutionary due to all its possibilities, its labyrinths, makes it a tool of extraordinary flexibility.

The description of this group of girls and boys reminded me of a scene I saw this morning before the door as I was waiting to smoke a cigarette. There was a lady with a puppy on a leash which jumped up and down between people's legs with immense joy and energy. This very picture seems to me to reflect the operation of this group. And this makes me also think of why adult patients find it so hard to deal with emotionality. The picture of this puppy, so evidently fond of its owner, makes me consider how once, a long time ago, these dogs were aggressive wolves ready to tear anybody to pieces; now though they have turned into puppies. These boys too, these other 'puppies', were raised to become and live like wolves, but at your centre they have been humanised precisely owing to the work of the educators.

This is the third or fourth time we have discussed in our seminars the work of the street educators and every time I am delighted. 'Time, work and passion' are the three keywords. Do you want a logo? A flag! Here you go! . . . And forget about the municipal orders!'

My impression is that you should get rid of the bureaucratic structure, of the Ethics Committee: then secondly get rid of all the elitist structures and finally all the hierarchic ones. Naturally this is extremely difficult to realise: the fear of chaos is always too strong and spreads like a true plague, which raises the question of the role of the media. I myself made various experiments in that direction which all resulted in failure. For instance, my attempt at creating a means of communication, of sharing information without a hierarchic structure or an elitist way of operation behind it, was a failure and burnt out on its own due to the lack of interest from those who were part of the experiment. Another attempt was to devise a new organisation modelled on the School of Athens; this experiment also failed because the people at the end wanted a qualification, a diploma. The inevitable consequence of a work group is individualism and hence solitude.

So if we first said the motto is 'time, work and passion', we can now add to this triad 'solitude'.

The value system that is naturally being fought against, against which perhaps nothing can be done because it is indestructible, is based on the notion of 'success'. I don't know if there is a way to measure or assess success, and this fact leads to the still so controversial question of statistics. Of all the art forms the only one which has a successful organisation is perhaps music: there is no other art form able to organise the work of so many persons as in an orchestra. The reason why no other art form can equal the successful organisation of music is because no other art form has a system of notes which allows artists to collaborate with colleagues without solitude. The musical notation is extraordinary and means that music can be taught to very young children with significant results. Any other art form, though, is bound to be taught only through example.

A seminar like this one also reflects perfectly the principle I'm seeking to demonstrate, because we too can learn only by means of an example. The reason for this, in my view, has to do once again with the fact that words by themselves do not offer a true notational system. The sole worthwhile element in verbal speech is apparently the lexical meaning, which however may result in a variety of ambiguities. Therefore the meaning of the words we pronounce should be sought not in the words alone but in the musicality they contain, where is manifest what we actually wish to express and communicate. We are not saying but showing it. And this is precisely the strength of the educators in this social service NOH: their ability to demonstrate, the example they offer, the passion they invest in their work.

Now you might ask me: 'Why don't they then just chat away, if in the end it's the same thing?' The fact is in practice this is what they are just doing! To get an idea of what it means to get rid of musicality of words, just try to talking with an obsessive neurotic.

Now going back to the earlier question about how to transform a way of thinking founded on basic assumptions into one of a work group, the answer could be to start looking into basic functions. The method we're employing here now is the only one I know for teaching psychoanalysis, or that of 'singing to one another' our clinical experiences. Because the moment we move away from clinical experience, all the words become a chatter, empty and useless jargon. This report by the street educators, by contrast, abounds in anecdotal clinical material. In psychoanalysis, the training is personal analysis. The usual question goes 'but how and when does it end?' It never does.

Wittgenstein offers a very interesting and appropriate example for teaching mathematics, showing that there is no way to imagine a highly complex series of numbers other than through intuition; it's like when a light bulb turns on suddenly and the student tells the teacher: 'I've got it, now I can go ahead and continue with the series.' But he knows it only intuitively, only like this does he understand the work method. The problem with intuitive thinking and progress is the moment when someone asks: ' But how did you do it?', and you have to reply: 'through intuition'. Naturally someone who does not think intuitively won't accept this, nor will he ever understand this kind of answer. Similarly, a small child can hardly believe he could learn to play a musical instrument; he might think, for instance, if someone has managed to play the piano he's done so by a stroke of luck, by chance, trying to bang on the keys until all of a sudden music came out of it. Once I heard a tape recorded by an autistic child who had never had piano lessons yet who could simply give life to musical compositions on the piano. Likewise, I happened to study the case of another autistic child who only needed to look at a building for few minutes to take up pen and paper and draw it in great detail and precision. What do such examples mean? That the human brain can potentially do an innumerable series of wonderful things. So what happens to the faculty of intuition which we all have? And why doesn't it develop? I'd venture to state that this faculty instead of developing is destroyed as we become subject to the educational process imposed by our school system.

Participant: Yet among those potential factors there is also the one that causes chaos: there are also destructive impulses, not only positive ones.

DM: You say this because you assume chaos is a negative thing. Everybody fears chaos. By definition chaos is a random thing, a thing of chance that has no meaning. But perhaps there's nothing that may be considered entirely deprived of significance, as is the case of chance; we are simply faced with ignorance, and lack of imagination and creativity.

I'd like to give the same answer as before to explain the passage from basic assumption mentality to that of the work group: first of all single out the areas of rigidity, then get rid of them. I imagine it would be very difficult to do analysis without knowing who the next patient is, when he's coming, without getting paid, without setting time limits, without considering that a day is made of 24 hours and that you can't work without a break. The best thing probably would be to start with acknowledging one's own impotence and vulnerability.

Participant: As regards intuition, it certainly is a mysterious concept; but what you are saying seems to suggest that there are ways of distinguishing the mental attitudes which can nourish intuition. For example, evoking something could be a mental process that might help develop intuition. When working in a sort of psychoanalytic cineforum, for instance, we ask the group to recall certain film scenes and at the end by putting them together we are able to trace the sort of mental operation enacted through that film.

DM: The way I see it is: intuition is something that can be stimulated simply by accepting the condition of submission with regard to an internal process over which one has no control.

Participant: I've formed an idea of intuition as something that exists but is kept silent about as it is regarded culturally as less 'professional' than rational planning.

DM: I cannot but agree with you.

CHAPTER THREE

Avoiding the Oedipus complex
(2001)

Giuseppina Pavan

I n April 1988 a colleague who works in a community for drug addicts asked me if I could take into psychotherapy one of her patients who had recently come out of the community after being under her care for some months. She believed it was important for her patient to have a therapist who was not in direct contact with the community and who pursued a psychodynamic approach.

The first session with Sarah

Sarah comes wearing a pair of sports trousers and track shoes. She is 34, has long beautiful hair and an interesting face; she avoids looking at me directly. The tone of her voice remains unvaried, as though she were trying not to show her feelings; even to date she continues talking in this monotonous voice.

She says she suffers from anxiety, adding: 'I left the community in November and am still seeing the doctor.'

When I ask her to talk about herself, Sarah makes a long list of her difficulties: 'At seventeen I became anorexic; then at 23 I started "doing it" occasionally, but went on to massive doses when I moved to Rome for work. At 30 I went back home. At 27 I met a boy who I soon discovered was HIV positive; for four years I had regular blood tests to make sure I wasn't positive myself. In the meantime I got carcinoma in the womb but did nothing about it: I was too worried about AIDS. I also had hepatitis C. I drank, got drunk, and shot heroin. I went in and out of the alcoholism departments of various hospitals, all in vain. At that point I joined the community and stayed there for two years, and it made me feel well; now I still fancy a shot but less so, and despite the depression I manage to restrain myself. I'm afraid of falling back on it, of not being able to live on without the community. I'd be fine on a train; I really don't know where to live. I'd like to be independent from my family, though I am not. I have rented a house in Trieste; my boy friend wants to live with me but I don't know what I want. I studied design at the Art School. In Rome I worked in an advertising agency where I was appreciated. At 30 I had a serious depression. First they fired me because the agency wasn't doing well; then I was employed again as I was good at my job. I could stand it a month: just worked and did nothing else, and then started shooting heroin again.'

I ask her about her family.

'My father never showed me any love. The only thing he said when I turned seventeen was I could not stay out. I hate my parents but am also happy to be with them. I have similar feelings towards Federico, who left the community with me: I want to be with him but then realise I don't want to. Now I see my sister Gianna and Aldo, a friend where I work part-time; I don't earn much. I was raised by my father's mother. She died when I was twelve or thirteen and left me in deep grief. This caused me to menstruate; I told no one and pretended nothing had happened. No one noticed my grief except my sister Gianna. My sister Luisa, herself a doctor, is better off than the two of us. Gianna is about to give birth and has come to live with my parents again. My mother has changed: now she is more helpful. My father though has always been tough. I show them that I am independent and need nothing, but it is not true at all. I fear I may no longer do the job I like or lose my boyfriend. I fear I've wasted a lot of time and that it is now too late to do anything. I still don't know whether I actually left the community or not. At first I said nothing, almost nothing about myself. I didn't talk to others, and doing it now is very trying.'

The third session

During this session Sarah tells me a dream: *She was in a bar offering drinks to friends and had a train to catch. There were some men and women but she knew none except Luca. She didn't know what station it was; she had to get on the train but the bartender was busy doing something else and she couldn't pay; this way she missed the 19.00 train.*

She told me her associations: 'I had no idea where the train was going, but I was very angry although I did know it wasn't because of the bartender that I missed the train – a woman I can't describe properly, roughly 38 years old. I used to go to the Art School on the 19.00 train. But didn't know where I was and where I was going. I nearly always buy drinks for others when I go out with friends. I can't stand not following the rules and want to plan everything. Luca comes from Udine, where my parents live. He invited me to go out for a pizza but I don't want to mess up. He used to take drugs, I don't know if he is still on drugs now. At Udine I see only my parents and my sister, but I don't want to live there; I'd be under their control, and as I don't know how to be independent I always need others. I seek Federico's protection when I want to keep away from my parents; I don't wish to remain alone.'

I find myself reflecting that the bartender, although younger than myself, might be me who prevents her from going to a place where she used to feel at ease and that I want her to stop and think about her difficulties.

After the first three sessions she tells me she wants to continue. I stress that this will be a beginning while she herself regards it as a continuation; she is in great anxiety and has wept a lot. When she comes to the sessions she sometimes thinks she may stay on with her family in Udine, where she currently works`; 'I don't know if there is room for me after my niece's birth.' Her sister has given birth and is now living with the parents. Sarah says: 'To begin here with you in this city seems to me like going back', adding: 'I fear I may go on heroin again if I no longer see the previous doctor.'

History

Sarah's mother is 68 years old and is a headmistress. Her father, 76, is a retired arts teacher and enjoys drawing as a hobby. Sarah is their third daughter. Her eldest sister Luisa, older by six years, is a doctor, married with an eight-year-old daughter. The other sister Gianna is two years older than her and teaches humanities; she lives with her partner and has recently had a baby girl.

Sarah says her mother has always been away from home; her father though has always been with them and has been very strict. Her mother used to earn more than her father; she kept the family going. At times the parents had a tense relationship and the father hit her mother several times. As a child, she used to spend the Christmas holidays with her father's mother, while the rest of the family left for the south, where her mother's mother lived. At Easter, though, it was her turn to head south with her mother.

Sarah explains that as a child she had to follow her sister Gianna, that is she was forced to do the things her sister enjoyed doing after school 'so that her mother could spare time'. She went to a religious elementary school run by nuns and had to have special attention from an assistant teacher as she was too reserved and taciturn. When they became teenagers her father wouldn't allow the sisters to go out with their friends or to invite them to their home.

After completing high school with excellent marks, Sarah went to art school and finished her studies. She talks of her university years as a period of great happiness and physical growth: she became rounder with hair dyed platinum blonde, wore high heels and skirts even in the winter, and was surrounded by friends of both sexes. At 20 she had an abortion.

After earning her university degree she left for Rome to work in an important advertising company directed by Una, a very successful and attractive woman. She shared a flat with two girls from her own hometown but they did not work and enjoyed an easy life; later though she moved to a flat above Una's. In Rome she felt utterly lonely. She regularly used heroin and drank heavily. For two and a half years she had a relationship with a man much older than herself, a drug addict. She lost her job due to work shortage at the agency, but soon was called back and her skills were put to good use again. For a year and half she kept drinking and having serious anxiety crises, during which she'd lock herself in and simply lie in bed. She could regain her peace of mind only when admitted to hospital. After her admission to the alcoholism department, her older sister moved her to her own house and to a different alcoholism centre. Sarah, however, continues to feel ill.

Her older sister's friends suggested she should enter the drug rehabilitation centre where she met Federico and established a stable relationship with him.

Donald Meltzer: She is strikingly restless but does not seem to be irritable. This kind of restlessness, particularly in adolescence, usually goes along with great irritability and a progressive paranoid-type withdrawal. She doesn't seem to be irritable and her withdrawal does not seem to be very paranoid. Her family attachments are strong but ambivalent; her relationships with men seem insubstantial and fraught with some sort of anxiety, particularly the fear of AIDS with Federico. Her emotional attachments seem fairly restricted to her family life. She is very group oriented; and it looks as though it has a rather addictive quality, being dependent and ambivalent, and easily led by other girls in particular.

She has certainly poured out a lot of information to the therapist and it seems to imply a desire to be known that indicates her loneliness.

The first year of therapy

Sarah is initially worried I may not take her on; she is afraid of not pleasing me; she talks but keeps her distance. She says she is angry with Federico, something she cannot tell him, for he has changed, he is no longer protective towards her as he was at the community, he has become aggressive and now insults her. She thinks she has never felt well and cannot stay well on her own. She lives in Trieste now, where the community is located, in a single-room flat with Federico; he pays no rent, saying his pay for the time being is not enough. Her father too used to earn less than her mother and spent her money as if it had been his. All the men she has had a relationship with have always been aggressive, insulting her just like her own father, and drug addicts.

After she has been coming to the sessions for some time she still complains that she does not know whether she can count on me, whether I'll be there for her. At times she wonders and fears she has arrived at the wrong time, something which has in fact never occurred.

She paid a visit to the family house at the seaside where she hadn't been for three years. At seventeen she started taking (sniffing) heroin there. Sarah adores the sea, especially the sea in southern Italy, and loves sunbathing. In the summer she takes off her clothes and feels physically much better. She is very anxious about my own holidays.

The agency where she works is again in difficulty and she risks losing her job again. A young colleague, Laura, suggests opening their own agency but she hesitates. While I was away on holiday, she says she had a difficult month, yet could get to sleep without feeling anxious and even read a book, something she hadn't done for a while. She seems to be happy to see me back from holidays, although she keeps a significant distance and talks in her usual monotonous voice.

She looks for a job in Trieste and in September finds one as a graphic designer in an advertising company. The new director is an extremely ill-tempered woman who insults her but appreciates her work. Now Sarah wonders whether she should continue the therapy in Udine. She accuses me of being 'an abstract entity' for her. This is precisely how she used to perceive her mother: 'I could only count on my grandmother, she liked me, but my mother wasn't there for me.' In fact I too doubted whether we could establish a good relationship that would allow us to work together. At times I did feel she was too distant, and I reacted by distancing myself, and often had to force myself to pay careful attention to what she was telling me. I tried to create a reassuring and stable situation at a very slow pace, never imposing a rigid setting. This is why, after getting a new job in Trieste, she comes only once a week; though later she asks to come twice. She fears I may think she is worthless, something she felt as a child. She still feels treated as a child. At the same time she feeds my doubts about my own capacity and the possibility of getting closer to her to help her.

In the city where she works, her work contacts are minimal; she is in touch with Laura, her younger colleague. She complains about Federico but she admits not being able to imagine living without him. She feels empty inside, adding 'it was usually when I felt like this that I went on heroin.' However, she manages to stick to her work; she thinks she is underpaid but also knows she is learning useful things for her profession. At this company she is asked to take on more responsibility than in Rome.

When I get back from the Christmas holidays, she tells me she has missed me. She received a car as a Christmas present from her mother; now she drives between Udine and Trieste. She sees her body as weak and does not look after it as she used to when at college. She thinks all her life now 'revolves around' work and the rest is in a mist. She also admits no longer liking Trieste. She begins to consider herself no longer a patient of the community.

Then her father has a stroke, goes into a coma and dies within two days. Federico goes to Sarah's house in Udine for the first time. Sarah now suffers a lot, saying: 'They told me I was my father's favourite daughter, perhaps because I'm an artist. He [my father] told me to go on, not to turn back.'

She spends a month at her mother's; she wants to make sure that her mother is doing well and that she also doesn't die. She buys a bathing suit and dreams of her mother now as a happy woman, freed from her father.

Federico asks her to buy a house of their own and marry him.

The second year of therapy

Insecurity continues to invade everything: 'I don't know where to live, what to do. My mother sent me a million lire and I don't feel like buying a house with that money. I just want to get away from it all.' Her sister Luisa gets drunk more regularly and Gianna does not leave their mother's house. She goes to the seaside with Federico and her mother; she dreams that *her mother comes into the room she is in with Federico, gets angry with her and throws her out.* Her longing to stay close to her mother and earn the place of the only daughter by her side contrasts with her relationship with Federico.

She now makes up her mind to quit her job in Trieste and open her own agency with Laura, younger but less experienced than herself. For the time being she works from home in Trieste and from her mother's house. She perceives both Federico and her mother as intruders in her life; the former uses her things, even her computer, and the latter simply overwhelms her.

Her mother offers boarding to college students; this makes her jealous as they occupy the study and she has to move to another room to work. Moreover, every time she comes to Udine, her sister Gianna comes for a visit too.

DM: It makes her sound very obsessional; but actually it is not a matter of obsessionality but of confusion. Her attachment to her father seems to be a very infantile one; and the dream that her mother is happy now her father is dead, seems to be about herself: that she is free from that attachment to her father. She finds any attachment really burdensome.

This fundamental situation in her character is now taking shape in the transference, in the form of her being very difficult to make contact with, and maintaining a position of distance and distrust toward the therapist. This uncertainty about the therapist seems to centre on the separations, which she doesn't tolerate very well; in so far as this is really a preformed transference rather than an operational transference, it seems to have been shifted directly from her mother. In a certain sense it is very challenging, but the therapist, like Federico, is always on trial (is he good enough for her). It brings into focus her grandiosity, which she calls being 'a bit of an artist' – 'being good at it'. This seems to imply that she is naturally talented: not something she has to work at, or a function of her interest, but just that it is in her nature to be talented. How much this grandiosity is attached to her body is uncertain, although the dreams suggest she considers her body to be compellingly attractive. (She buys herself a bathing suit and dreams of her mother being happy.)

She seems to pass up opportunities, like the one of forming a partnership with Una, or to make any sort of relationship with Federico. This general aspect of a drug addict personality depends greatly on sensuality and comfort. The sensuality is at very animal level, like a cat that can't find a comfortable position unless it is in the sun. She doesn't have sustained attachments. She is not searching for a relationship so much as offering herself for a relationship, and sitting in judgement on the people who are attracted to her – whether physically or because of her talents is very nebulous. What is noticeably lacking is any infrastructure, any evidence for her having an interest in anything in particular. She isn't interested in money, status, relationships, sex – it's all at a much more nebulous sensual level. She is probably more gratified by a group situation than by any individual relationship. These group situations are not relationships but a network of acquaintanceship that involves a kind of parasitism. Her so-called friends are people on whose floors she can sleep, for whom she buys drinks or drugs when they are together, and whose behaviour she mimics as a group member. The network is treated as a safety-net.

It doesn't even satisfy her need for security but only a kind of myth of security: she doesn't need a house because she feels she has access to all these houses where she can sleep, have a bath, and so on.

So we are talking really about an unacknowledged form of parasitism, a very primitive form of sensuality. What is interesting from a therapeutic point of view would be to scout out her grandiosity, which I think centres on this combination of physical beauty and presumed artistic talent.

Shall we continue.

GP: Sarah no longer stays silent with Federico and she gets angry; he is finding it increasingly difficult to get on with her. They are both jealous. She's thinking of opening her own studio in Udine and wants it to be like mine. She also says: 'At my mum's I'm almost better than in Trieste. We have dinner at 9 pm, watch TV, without really following it, and I sit in my father's place.' Gianna asks her mother if she can live in her house, rather than buying a flat for herself. In this case there'd be no room left for Sarah. Jokingly she adds that 'she'll only have me.'

She also starts reflecting on her work experience in Rome, where Una prevented her from speaking her mind and used to order her around which she went along with. Now she says she no longer likes some of Una's work.

Shortly before the anniversary of her father's death, she comes to know from her relatives that she won't come into any money, for together with her sisters she has signed an agreement to leave all his estate to her mother to avoid paying high taxes. And on her mother's death, only the grandchildren will be the entitled heirs and as Sarah has no children, she will inherit nothing. Her mother offers to buy her a house to make up for the loss. But she says no, adding it is not only a matter of money. She feels she is the last and the least provided for.

She then relates a dream in which *she was in a crowded place getting something to eat and her new bag suddenly disappeared with all the money, papers and bankcard. She got angry. The police came; then she saw herself drunk, confused, and everyone came and went as though it was a hostel.* She says she is tempted now and again to go back on heroin. She dreams of sniffing it, has a good reserve of it but thinks she should first talk about it with me. The work we are doing together has gained more substance.

Some recent sessions

The first session of the week

Sarah is worried about what has happened in the US [the Twin Towers]. Afterwards she says she had a different weekend than usual; she spent it at the seaside with a friend, a girl she'd recently met in Trieste who wanted to do something together with her. Federico, who usually does not bother to ring her when she is in Trieste and goes after his own business, this time round rang her several times on her mobile. They went out with friends on Sunday, but Federico got bored and left for home, then went to a friend's house in the evening and got back home in the morning; nevertheless she slept on.

Then her thoughts turn to her work; she is now very busy but fails to get paid on time. Then she thinks about her mother who is not well and about her sister Gianna, who seems to have disappeared since her new house was finished. While she was in Trieste her other sister Luisa, going through a deep crisis, went to stay a couple of days at their mother's house.

Sarah is no longer interested in the idea of having her own flat and her constant wavering makes her laugh. She then tells of her recent bad dreams; in one of these *an acquaintance informs her that some people are cheating her and that she needs to defend herself; she gets angry and fires them.* She also adds that this acquaintance is someone who brings in work for her; 'he offered certain commissions from one of his clients whom he himself had recommended to me, but this client happens to be the client of a rival company so I refused the work; I cannot work with a rival company.' In another dream she *wanted to talk about herself with her sister Luisa, but she heard her talking to her husband about her on the phone in a derogatory way. She hung up and didn't call her.* She says her sister Luisa is now divorcing her husband, is not well, and she doesn't know how to help her: 'It was always Luisa who helped me; I don't think she can actually talk badly about me to her husband.'

I try to draw Sarah's attention to the fact that a part of herself may be cheating her, may be attacking her, and that nurtures bad intentions; but Sarah does not reply.

The second session of the week

She says she is feeling 'heavy', so I ask her why. She says: 'I'm not happy with anything. Today I was thinking what would happen if Federico and I were to split; I kept aloof so I could think about it. Last night, always on the phone as he never wishes to discuss things when we are together, he asked me what I thought about our relationship. I think there are so many things that do not work, but I don't have enough energy to deal with them. He said he finds me annoying in Trieste as he has his friends and interests, while I have nothing but my job.'

I remind her that last Saturday she went out with a friend; she replies she 'only followed her'. Sarah then says: 'I fail to see a future, and just live day by day, which makes me really sad and feel lonely.'

Now Sarah is less concerned with Federico and more centred on herself. She says: 'My friends asked me to go to the cinema with them in the evening; a film they have made will be shown, so I'm going.'

I say she finds it difficult to admit being interested in it herself too.

'Yes', says Sarah, 'it does interest me but I can hardly bring myself to express it. I can hardly take an initiative: I could go to the gym, right across from my mother's house, but I don't. It is difficult to make decisions. There is my work, but that too has gone stale. I could be satisfied with my work; yesterday I was praised for presenting a product, my name will be on it. It is comfortable to spend some time in Trieste and some in Udine, so I don't dig deeply into things.'

I point out that Udine for her means not only her family but also her work and the therapy, while Trieste stands for Federico and that it may not be too easy for her to keep these two parts of herself together.

She says: 'I envy Federico for doing what pleases him; I feel sterile and alone. Winter is approaching and I am feeling ugly and old. Others are dressed better than me; I have nothing, I must buy something. Soon it's my birthday, I'll turn 37, I dread it; I feel lonely. The girl friend I went out with last Saturday has just divorced after 20 years, and says now she is finding positive things about herself she didn't know she had. But she also says she hates families. I don't want to get consumed like this. I feel sterile, approaching 40 and I have relationships only with other people's sons.'

Discussion

GP: On the countertransference level I perceive her as a burden, yet at the same time I have come to like her very much.

DM: There are endless rather psychopathic goings on in this network of friends who continually exploit one another, tell lies and talk behind one another's backs. It is a terrible climate, this network.

It is easy to confuse the claustrophobia that accompanies membership of a group such as this with processes of projective identification; but in fact it doesn't involve identification at all. It involves this very loose web of mutual exploitation, dissembling and so on.

GP: I also think so, I don't know if it is true but that's what I think as well.

Participant: It seems the patient is trying to draw in the therapist to feeling sorry for her.

DM: It is a type of preformed transference, taking the form of a direct repetition of the child's relationship with her mother at the borderland of puberty and adolescence: when the mother's home is used simply as a place for bringing friends home and conducting sexual explorations, and the mother at her wits' end.

Participant: How old was she when she started taking drugs?

GP: Seventeen. She is now 37.

Participant: So she is still seventeen. She has missed the next 20 years.

DM: The significance of group membership doesn't depend on the type of group: it could be an army, a social group, a delinquent group, a religious group. The consequences are the same: a sacrifice of development. One meets patients whose lives have been wasted in opportunism, and this always involves their 'friends', but the friends keep changing: last year's friends become unfriendly today.

The way to get at the transference is to represent the analytic situation as an analytic family, and to refuse to treat it as a network group. This involves being fairly strict with the patient about their demands and expectations of being indulged. Of course you have to put up with accusations that you are aloof, don't treat her as a daughter, are just out for the money and so forth. Endless abuse: not of a claustrophobic type, just the abuse of a street urchin in being excluded from family life.

It is only by exploring this resentment of being excluded from the family that you get anything like an Oedipus complex that doesn't consist simply of being daddy's favourite, having parents who are estranged or know nothing of one another, in which mummy and daddy are just part of the network of middle-aged people who are in power and control the money – a completely social and political attitude that excludes any possibility of the true Oedipus complex.

With the Oedipus complex, there are always more babies to come. You can see it in the description of her mother's big house which is constantly filled with tenants or visitors – the patient can't stand all these new babies coming along. And that is the transference situation.

She expected her father's death would be a relief not only to her mother but also to herself. But it hasn't turned out that way. So it's not surprising that it becomes so difficult to keep contact with the transference as soon as there is a holiday break.

CHAPTER FOUR

A potential terrorist: the conflict with anti-life forces
(2002)

Elena Pianezzola

I thought of bringing this case to Dr Meltzer's attention because I don't know how to pursue the therapy of this young girl; at times I have the feeling that between us there are only words and that these do not translate into an emotional bond, so this will consequently thwart the possibility of growth too.

I have been seeing Emma for two sessions a week for the past two years from the age of 25. She has two elder brothers: Giacomo, age 30, who is autistic, and Gilberto, age 27. Her mother is a retired teacher and her father is an accountant. To get her degree in Education Sciences, Emma still has to pass a good number of exams, do an apprenticeship period and write her final dissertation; but currently she is blocked, unable to pursue and conclude her studies.

She is a nice looking, fragile girl. With her very fair skin and long dark chestnut hair she resembles a porcelain statue both in the way she looks and the way she moves. She speaks in a monotonous voice quite rapidly and has a slightly foreign accent.

At our first meeting I ask about her problems and symptoms and she explains:

> **Emma:** I have come to you because I have a problem: my hair is thinning, a form of androgenic alopecia; this is very important for me and gives me great pain. Because of this I went to see a dermatologist who prescribed a few tests. As well as that I have another problem, blood microcirculation disorder; I feel my stomach closes up, I eat very little yet feel heavy all the time. The dermatologist asked me to do these tests and also suggested I be treated psychologically.
>
> Well, I do know the way I relate to my hair is not normal; I spend a lot of time and attention on my hair care, but I do not know if this could explain my hair loss or help prevent it. I know all this care amounts to no good but I can do nothing else. I also have difficulty communicating with others and realise it's getting worse. I am very unhappy; I see this unhappiness is ruining my life and making me withdraw further into myself. There are other problems too like feeling tired, at times I can barely lift my arms.
>
> My hair began thinning about a year and a half ago, in August. It's been slow but progressive. I am also losing eyelashes and eyebrows; tests at the time gave good results – that is it wasn't a matter of hormone imbalance, which would have been worse. The hair loss I had was quite marked, and then it's concentrated on a certain spot – here in the middle of my forehead. I know thinking constantly so much about my hair sounds trivial and superficial but I am not superficial. My true nature is not like this, but I cannot help it; I am always so worried and unhappy.
>
> When I decided to study Education Sciences, I thought I would enjoy it; but as I went on it gradually dawned on me I might not be a suitable educator because you need strength to become one and I have none.

My feeling from this first interview was that Emma was a highly unhappy person, but there was also a marked rigidity in her as if she feared I might not be able to discover the possible reasons for her suffering, similar to the medical tests that produced no physical cause for her hair thinning; yet at the same time I felt she would be difficult to help, that it would be difficult to get at her. There is something conclusive about the way she presents herself which sounds like: 'That's it, there is no other viewpoint, no other way to see things.' We agree to meet again and make an appointment accordingly.

The second meeting

Emma begins by saying she is 'dead tired' owing to all her medical tests; she has been to a number of specialists: an endocrinologist, a dermatologist, and recently a gynaecologist.

Emma is very impatient about finding a solution to her problems, and cannot bear all these failed attempts to find a cure. While speaking she lays her hand at the top of her stomach, where she says she feels the internal weight, and continues:

> **Emma:** Now my anxiety has grown immensely as I think this disorder will be a sort of hallmark of my personality and will determine it without the least possibility of a change. I have never been a strong person, I've always been fragile and now that my hair is falling out I think the thing is settled. Whilst I regarded it as some internal fragility I could put up with it, but now it is visible to others I can no longer tolerate it. At college there were others with this thinning problem but they looked cheerful and self-confident; I always thought they were duping everyone while in actual fact they must be feeling very bad and were truly fragile, and now that mine has become visible I see no way out; besides I think I also have eating problems.
>
> **Therapist:** Why don't you eat?
>
> **Emma:** Well, I usually don't eat much, say, little and often. Now though I can no longer eat properly, I prefer savoury stuff, no sweets. I often prepare a dish of pasta which is so filling that I can eat no fruit or vegetables – there is no more room, not because I don't like them; mid afternoon I have a sandwich.
>
> **Therapist:** Who does the cooking at home?
>
> **Emma:** Mum, but recently it has become difficult for me to join the others at table.

Emma adds she has a sensation of freezing around her when in company with others and that she talks about superficial things. When I ask what things, she replies 'Music, cinema'. It is difficult for me to form an idea of Emma either as a cinema-goer or as a keen music listener.

> **Therapist**: You tell me you are very anxious but would you have sought psychological treatment had it not been for your hair loss?
>
> **Emma**: Probably not.
>
> **Therapist**: Who would you have talked about your problems with?
>
> **Emma**: With my mother because she had problems similar to mine and she understands me.
>
> **Therapist**: Did your mother have problems with thinning hair?
>
> **Emma**: No, it wasn't her hair, but certain states of anxiety, so she understands me very well.
>
> **Therapist**: Does your mother know that you are consulting a psychologist?
>
> **Emma**: My mother does, not my father, he doesn't understand and I don't want him to worry, I didn't even talk to him about my hair.

I tell her that in my view starting psychotherapy treatment would be beneficial, for I'm beginning to realise Emma is withering; her search for some physical cause, so far so fruitless, appears to be distancing the rescue buoy further from her reach. I tell her she needs to find a personal point of reference to initiate her treatment, a point that can link with all the various problems she is experiencing as a whole. Emma agrees, and to tell the truth does not even discuss the contract in detail, all in line with her manner of not lowering herself to inquire about prices and timetables.

Donald Meltzer: This is a sort of perversion of exhibitionism, in which Emma thinks that everything she thinks and does shows socially and other people respond to it, which humiliates and make her anxious. Apart from her mother who, she feels, understands her state of anxiety. What it is about her mother that exempts her from being an object of such anxiety is not clear. What the mother seems to understand is that Emma cannot tolerate her relationship with her father, and Emma separates them in her mind by making her father mindless.

One of the results of this splitting of the combined object is that she cannot eat with any pleasure. Correspondingly she has seen many specialists but she cannot really cooperate with anyone in any type of therapy. It is not only that nobody understands except her mother, but also her pessimism that there is nothing to be done. So it is very significant what she admits at the end: that she is the kind of person who never yields to negotiate questions such as prices and times. What she doesn't admit is how unyielding she is – she is just going her own way, like a buoy drifting off into the ocean as the therapist describes it. She is letting herself drift away from relationships.

Diagnostically we can say that the focal point of her character order is her negativism. The principle of negativism is fundamentally delinquent: a position is taken in which it is always the other person who has to prove something to them. And of course it is not possible to *prove* anything. As a technique of projecting rage into other people, it is a winner. It works every time. Rage is projected and people give up: they turn from trying to help her to battling her, reassuring her, being effusive and so on.

We know from experience of the world how useless negotiation is. Negotiation requires both sides being willing to change. You can see it creates a countertransference problem of incipient violence, as the therapist is beset with violent feelings towards the patient and her negativism. This is probably the same position that the father is placed in: being kept ignorant, denigrated and put to one side, left with feelings of rage and helplessness.

The problem of pessimism is a terrible one because it does give rise to feelings of murderousness in other people. The key to it is the belief in the efficacy of punishment: which of course leads one directly into the trap of the patient's masochism – that they will invite punishment. The countertransference problems are terrific really. The therapist's opportunities for punishing the patient are limited almost exclusively to throwing her away, which would be perfect gratification for her masochism. 'I don't want to worry my father' – where worrying is treated as if it were synonymous with being aroused to murderousness.

So far it looks like an intractable problem, because of the pessimism and the masochism underlying it. The thing that has to be tackled with a patient like this, which will arouse her violence, is the implication that she enjoys her omnipotent negativism. She enjoys torturing other people.

When you study problems of masochism you find inevitably that their problems are actually of sadism; and the object of their sadism is always the next baby: it is the killing of babies. The evidence for this is always to be found in their dreams. The killing of babies is so much a part of our culture that it passes unnoticed really. The murderous meaning is hidden in all sorts of social rituals.

We are at the beginning of the therapy; and the therapist has little choice but to wait to see what happens. You have been warned that she is the sort of person who never negotiates.

Beginning of the therapy

The unchanging principal feature of the sessions is that Emma starts talking as soon as she lies down on the couch, taking up her speech at the same point she left off the previous time as if she and I have never separated. Even her tone of voice remains the same, carrying only slight emotional variations; she displays no curiosity, no interest, asks no questions, and makes no comments about me. I am simply there, which at times makes me feel like one of the pictures hanging on the wall. Otherwise, as I once pointed out to her, I am no more than a big ear to listen attentively to all she has to say. The way she moves remains unvaried as well (even today she tends to walk in front of me rather than have me accompany her). The first year she'd lie down on the couch, ceremoniously unfasten her hair clip and put it back again at the end of the session, making me watch the elaborate show.

Following the very first session she introduces a delay of ten minutes to the time of the appointment: the sessions start at 3 pm but she shows up at 3.10. The various interpretations of this delay come to nothing; once she even says she enjoys having people wait for her!

At the beginning she was filled with so much anxiety that she felt like throwing up and as the session drew near she had to take tranquillizers. The weight she felt in her stomach stopped her from eating, or rather it took her a very long time, nearly two hours, to finish a meal. The others, her father and brothers, would get up and leave the table, while her mother sat with her to the end. She'd eat as instructed by the doctors to avoid growing weaker. Emma does not trouble herself in the least with housework; it is Gilberto who does the house duties like vacuum cleaning, and helping their mum with washing up.

At this period a boy called Davide asked to go out with her; however, as Emma is so worried and self-conscious about her hair, she'd only agree to go out when she was sure he hadn't noticed her thinning hair.

When on top of eating one adds the amount of time she requires to prepare before going out, all done in the bathroom, her entire day is spent in this fashion. She sleeps until late in the morning, stays in her pyjamas and never feels she has had a rest.

Emma behaves as if she were a 'beautiful statue'; never compares herself with her peers; rather, she is filled with a sort of self-idealisation which makes her at most gaze at models in glossy magazines; at times she even fancies the magazine model's hair is also thinning. Another characteristic of Emma's is that if she says in one session she feels blocked, ill at ease and so on, in the following session the focus returns to that point in order to shift the argument about her discomfort in her favour. Thus: 'Last time I said I wanted to be more relaxed, but that doesn't mean I enjoy being like those people who talk all the time. It is true I'm not very talkative but that doesn't mean I don't have deep thoughts, only that I wish I weren't so tense.'

In June, nearly after three months into therapy, Emma relates a dream about her relationship with Giacomo. It is a dream about a newborn baby: *There was a small baby, a newborn who I believe was a baby son of my parents, a beautiful baby lying in a cot with sides, like the white ones in hospitals, and I was looking at him and stroking his cheeks. Next to him I saw Giacomo and I had, for a very short time, a normal conversation with Giacomo. A very, very short but normal one. He was lying next to the newborn baby with an arm over the blanket (we were both as big as we are now), and at one point I noted the baby was no longer there; I was afraid and tried to call my parents, very worried because he was not under the blanket. I tried to put on the lights which wouldn't switch on, then my parents came and told me 'true, he is no longer there.' I said: 'But you made me believe there was a baby and now he's gone and I've told everyone about him!' They explain they were told to lead me to believe it, to pass the time.*

DM: She makes the baby disappear: particularly if they are beautiful babies. She is always changing her mind, her story: treating you as if you were a detective and throwing you off the scent of the murderer who has killed the baby.

EP: Emma has thought of making Giacomo disappear and might still be tormenting herself with the suspicion that she could have somehow contributed to his illness. Even today Emma does not communicate in any way with Giacomo, spares no time for him, doesn't go out with him and gets 'hysterical', in the words of her family, when Giacomo pulls her hair.

Emma's mother discovered Giacomo's autism when he was two years old, while expecting Gilberto. Emma 'discovered' her brother at nearly ten; before that, for her, Giacomo had been normal, no one at home had said a word about his illness. Emma and Gilberto have, between the two of them, nicknamed Giacomo 'the boss.'

DM: This is typical of autism, that the autistic child turns the parents into slaves; mother and father are at his service.

EP: After a few months, Emma decides to go back to her studies; she is neither convinced they will help her nor has much interest, but she wants to finish them. She's still going out with Davide and feeling low both when he calls her and when he fails to do so. Her relationship with her mother is still tightly knit; she confides in her every single state of her mind; moreover, she seems to enjoy a little seeing her mother put the blame on herself, for the latter believes she hasn't done enough for her children and is upset to see her offspring so unprepared for life. She also starts talking about her rancour-filled relationship with her father. In her view he is responsible for not having allowed her to lead a normal life like other girls. She couldn't go out because it was too dangerous (no bikes), or too silly (see all those idiots huddled under the umbrella on the beach), or too common and worthless; in fact he was constantly putting off allowing her to do anything until the day came when she could really understand things.

Her father usually asks her to have a drink. At home they have a wide choice of wines and spirits. All too often her father has a drink and asks Emma to join him so as not be left alone. Emma is irritated because of this service yet accompanies him. She is in contact with only three or four of her highschool friends, and with great difficulty responds to their invitations. At first such suggestions, even the ringing of the phone, disquiet her; later she simply refuses to join them by making up some excuse. If she ever accepts an invitation, she spends the evening without speaking, intensely edgy or critical, and back at home disappointment reigns.

The first summer break

I am very worried about the coming summer holiday, and afraid of appearing to be leaving Emma alone and helpless. She makes no holiday plans with Davide or her girl friends. She's tired of studying, does not even mention the prospect of a job; I, but not she, expect trouble is looming ahead. Indeed after the holidays, unfortunately, my fears prove true. She says she is feeling bad because she heard nothing from Davide; in mid-August she stayed in bed unable to stand on her feet and her parents were worried she might become anorexic.

A few days before I get back from holiday, she starts eating again, thinking it is due to Davide's call which has raised her spirits. She wishes to give up therapy, saying she has been too unwell and too disturbed to find herself so dependent on Davide. We get down to work, I decide to shoulder the weight myself, but Emma refuses to listen, adding she didn't miss the sessions. In the end, though, she concedes: 'The thing is when I tell you about Davide and you tell me that I am angry with Davide or you, well I might be a little bit, but the thing is this is not what I think …'.

DM: What the countertransference tells you is that suicide is present in everybody in relation to her and even in herself. Eventually somebody does kill themselves; in this case it will probably be Giacomo.

EP: In September after the holiday she tells me a dream she had in August:

Emma: In the dream *I was in a dining room and swimming, actually swimming-flying, for I hung in the air and drifted forwards and backwards like doing laps in a pool. My mum and my brother Giacomo were there too. She was seated on the old sofa which no one except Giacomo ever uses at home as it is completely sunken.*

Therapist: I think your swimming-flying in the air has to do with your keeping an eye on everything without ever setting foot on the ground; there are many interesting aspects in this dream, but to me the two poles are particularly important: the old sofa with Giacomo representing, say, 'no entry zone', and the new sofa which you always described as 'more comfortable'.

Emma: Now I remember another detail of the dream: I was a child, blonde with blue eyes, and my nose was bleeding. I often suffered from nosebleeds.

Therapist: Who has got blonde hair and blue eyes?

Emma: Davide.

Therapist: Any woman?

Emma: No, my mother has chestnut hair – dyes it red, though! At one time I also fancied having fair hair but not light-coloured eyes.

Therapist: When did your menstrual periods start?

Emma: At fourteen, accompanied by a terrible tummy-ache, terrible pains. This could be because no-one had ever told me a thing about it, I had no clue what was happening to me, I remember there were guests at home and I went to the bathroom where I actually threw up heavily, felt dizzy and had to take pills.

Therapist: How old was the child in your dream?

Emma: Seven or eight.

Therapist: And the child, what did she do with all that blood?

Emma: Nothing, she did nothing.

Emma endures the second summer break in 2001 better; nothing particularly nice occurs but at least she does not suffer as in the previous summer. I, on the other hand, experience a serious standstill towards her, finding it hard to move on, owing to Emma's narcissistic hair treatment which expands to dominate her entire being; her obsessive pondering, her repeated return to the same issues, increasingly make me doubt the likelihood of any headway. Emma says that at times she feels so tired of living that she rejoices to see her hair fall, like some sadistic joy at self-destruction. The winter passes without any emotional turbulence; I try not to turn into a life instruction manual for her, yet she keeps frustrating me by denying any emotional commitment while simultaneously turning to me for advice on how to live.

DM: Here we see a series of things that make us think of suicidal impulses or thoughts: her obsessive pondering, the repeated nosebleeds, even her sadistic pleasure at seeing her hair-fall. I think that the key to a problem like this is the very mysterious one of hallucination. When she changes her story told in the previous session it is because it is being dictated to her by a hallucinatory figure – what used to be called satanic possession, like a witch. She fills everybody with violence, murderousness, hatred, by the very simple device of negativism: a negativism that is dictated to her by an hallucinated voice.

The therapist is in despair about being able to effect any improvement in her inner claustrum. There is only one certain exit to the claustrum – and that is suicide. What these people do to those responsible for them is to wait for a moment when they are left alone to kill themselves and make everybody feel guilty about it. The essential thing about the hallucinatory voice is that it will tell this girl how and when to kill herself. It's not difficult to imagine the sense of relief and joy that ensues with such a person's disappearance; had it happened two hundred years ago children would also be invited to the party to see the witch burn (all this in line with maniacality). I'm thinking of Joan of Arc: when the saint's ghost appears and asks the crowd if they want her to return to life, the answer is 'no, absolutely no'.

Of course, psychoanalysts don't believe in the devil. But it's true that such an hallucinated voice does actually exist in certain patients, telling them what to do, what to say, how to behave. This dream of swimming and flying is a clear indication of the hallucinated suicidal urge which results in people killing themselves by throwing themselves out of the window with the idea that they could fly; it's not uncommon as the basis of this kind of psychopathology.

Participant: Is Dr Meltzer talking about a negative therapeutic reaction?

DM: The concept of the negative therapeutic reaction is a bit of a distortion really. It's turning the tables – when an analysis fails, who fails? Does the patient fail or does the analyst fail? Well I think the truth in such cases is that the analyst has failed to establish the analytic situation, that is, the communication of introspective observation. Patients who describe themselves from the outside are not cooperating in the analytic situation and there is simply no possibility of establishing an analysis with them. They just tell you chronicles, ready formulated stories.

Emma is a witch. The focal point is always the killing of the baby.

Last session before the summer break, 2002

Emma arrives ten minutes late as usual and starts talking right away:

> **Emma**: I'd like to tell you I did well at the two university exams and I'm very happy about this. My mum but also my father were satisfied. When I got home they congratulated me; but because of some silly thing, some mistake with the shopping, my mother turned bitter and began complaining, and my father in the end grew nervous and they insulted each other. When I went back home with such good marks the strangest thing was Gilberto's face: sweet, relaxed and saddened. This is odd to me, I'd have expected him to be more annoyed because of my good exam results.
>
> **Therapist**: I think you find it difficult to imagine yourself as someone who could respond to sweetness and the pleasure of giving pleasure.
>
> **Emma**: Yes.

> **Therapist**: Well, we'll talk about it after the holidays.
> **Emma**: Yes.

First session after the summer break, 2002

After the usual ten-minute delay, Emma greets me briefly yet lies down on the couch with a smile.

> **Emma:** When I come back from a meeting with my girl friends I always feel empty; I never know if this feeling makes me feel better or worse. For instance, last night (Sunday) I went out with Gilberto who had been to a party on Friday and found it nice, so we went there again on Sunday. We stayed at the party about an hour; Gilberto had heard that his own friends who had recently married were expecting a baby, everybody knew it as they had told everyone except him. At that point I had the feeling of emptiness and gave vent to my frustration at home. How come others who are no better than me and Gilberto are so happy and satisfied whereas Gilberto and I, the same age as others, are so utterly different. On top of all, Gilberto's boy friends and my girl friends are no extraordinary people, to be honest, they are even commoner than the two of us, and yet they hardly ever feel so disconnected, so isolated. What makes me angry, actually brings me to tears, is to see Gilberto speak with such tenderness and gentleness as he deals with and tries to understand a situation, whereas I feel furious. My mother and Gilberto say I envy him but I don't believe them.
> **Therapist:** I think, Emma, on Sunday evening you lost all ability to imagine yourself in my mind and must have found yourself totally alone and therefore got furious (which is why you couldn't understand Gilberto's gentleness). On the other hand, you waver between two modes: you regard me as a piece of background furniture, you walked in without even asking me how I was doing; you left me pale and now find me suntanned, yet put no questions as though you could spare no time for it and start talking as if it were any other Monday and so on. I must also say some part of you must have kept me with care during the summer, as when you

stayed in contact with your friends. Yet you insist on not wishing to establish any relationship with me: where I was, who I was with, you don't want to encounter the object (me) whilst experiencing pain for being forgotten.

Emma: These friends are also quite nice.

Therapist: And you insist on not wanting to see me.

Emma: For me it's difficult to cope with other people's personal matters.

DM: You really scolded her for treating you as an inanimate object. What did she actually do to you? She depersonalised you: treating you as a thing, as non-existent. You are filled with what she projects into you by her negativity. Fundamentally she is afraid of you killing yourself.

You won't win your argument with her. She told you at the very beginning that she is incapable of negotiating.

Session before the Christmas break, 2002

Emma says she wants to talk about a dream she had the night before which makes her remember other similar previous dreams where she had very short cropped hair or an entirely shaven head. She has never talked about them before.

Emma: *I win a holiday trip out of a croissant packet – a one-week holiday in the Bahamas – and immediately feel happy. It doesn't say when to go and I agree to arrange a date with the company. Then I start having doubts about the departure date. I don't want to leave on my own. Then the scene changes and I'm in Venice, in a gondola with a group of young people I don't know, and I have further doubts about going on this trip. Then in another scene in the dream I'm still in Venice, in a perfume shop. As I try on a sunblock cream I still have the feeling of being in this unknown person's company, then I look around and believe I see S and T [her girl friends], who are also going on the trip; actually everything's ready for the departure. Towards late afternoon I realise I'm not ready yet; I haven't packed but more importantly, haven't washed my hair and think I cannot do it anywhere else but at home. Then they call me to confirm my departure but I no longer want to leave; I don't know how* *to say this. I grow increasingly aware that it's due to my hair, well my suitcase too, but mainly my hair.*

It's Gilberto who often eats croissants, not me. My mother buys him the sort with low sugar content as he tends to eat a lot.

Therapist: It's unusual to come across a holiday in the Bahamas inside a croissant packet; usually they give away sweets to children. What are your friends doing?

Emma: S is studying hard for her degree, F and B are leaving for Paris. T might leave as well, she's the sort that doesn't miss a chance, she just grabs it and goes, S is going too … actually they are all leaving.

Therapist: What about you? Don't you think of planning a trip with your friends or getting ready to go somewhere?

Emma: Now I remember, B was also in the dream but he wouldn't leave. In the dream when asked whether he would be going he said no as he had made it clear from the start he wasn't sure, while I don't know how to say no.

Therapist: In fact this dream seems to be talking directly about your Christmas holidays and you seem to feel it impossible to substitute your usual bathroom rituals.

Emma: It's impossible for me to travel. My father has already started nagging about my relationship with S, saying we are going out too often.

Therapist: What does he say about S?

Emma: That we two girls are going out in search of men.

Therapist: What does he think is wrong with that?

Emma: I don't know, in my view he is being dishonest by saying such things to me, anyway one can't talk with him.

Therapist: This may well be so, but if you refuse to fight to move on you may indeed find yourself with cropped hair or a shaven head, that is if you don't make use of your own abilities.

DM: The voice that calls to ask her to confirm her participation, which she says she doesn't feel like doing, is in actual fact the voice of hallucination. The question arises whether or not she is a liar. There is a difference between lying and confabulating. She's a confabulator: she says anything that comes to her mind, and it is your problem to disprove it. It's the technique of the antisocial character: what they say is true unless somebody else can disprove it. Of course you never get the chance. When you try to follow her she is always doubling back and you feel she is making a fool of you, because you have believed what she said. But belief doesn't come into it. She doesn't have to believe anything she says. She just has to wait for it to be disproved by the other person.

EP: I'd like to mention another dream in which *she sent an anthrax pie to Bush* (the American president).

DM: She is a terrorist!

EP: In that dream there were a good number of lawyers who had to prove her culpability while she looked perplexed saying: 'Look what a mess I end up in! They want to blame me for something without knowing whether I actually did it or not.'

DM: The story about Pontius Pilate is that 'jesting Pilate says, what is truth?' and does not wait for an answer.

Participant: Perhaps it could be a good idea if they were to agree on a trial period to find out ways of establishing an analytical situation.

DM: Clearly patients like this are a danger to one's character as a psychoanalyst; because they do arouse such murderous feelings that you would vote to have them burned at the stake. When I said to a patient whom I'm afraid I hate that she is wasting her time and her money because she is incapable of establishing a psychoanalytic situation, she said 'I can't stop because I'll feel a failure.' I said, 'You are a failure. I am as well. We have failed to establish an analysis.'

There is a lesson to be learned about establishing the analytic situation, which is something Mrs Klein spelled out over and over again. The centre of the analytic relationship is truthfulness – not just the analyst's but the patient's as well. *Truthfully* – we have no way of knowing the truth. But that doesn't stop us from being truthful. It requires introspection: being able to look inside your mind and truthfully report what you observe there.

Ultimately it is the dreams that tell the truth. This dream about the anthrax packet tells the truth that she is a suicide bomber. And I think this voice that she hears announcing the people who will go on the trip is the satanic voice that instructs her.

The therapist says quite accurately that the patient wants her to be a manual of instruction: that is, as to how she should behave in order to be above suspicion of being a suicide bomber.

Participant: So what can you do – terminate the analysis?

DM: You can't do that without an adequate trial. You can't tell in advance what is going on in the patient's mind, you only learn with experience. They will not admit consciously to their destructive and suicidal parts. It is the dreams that will tell you the truth. It is necessary to try for several years to establish the analytic situation. Of course it is a danger to your own mental health.

CHAPTER FIVE

Between aridity and hope
(1993)

Annamaria Mariuccia

Two and half years ago, a colleague working in a public service asked me to take Chiara into therapy. When I first met her she was 20 and in her second year at university. She needed my help because she had difficulty being with others and by herself; she felt a lot of tension in her back and neck muscles. She had stopped going to university lectures, for being in company with others was too demanding, and had even thought of dropping out altogether, which her mother tried to dissuade her from doing. To appear cheerful and carefree she had tried to imitate an extroverted friend, but it cost her an immense effort to be different from how and what she actually was. She lived in fear of her continually recurring crises of depression.

The first crisis had occurred in March in her last year at high school, making her feel so tense that she could no longer write during the lessons. This impediment made her feel so awkward she could not tell anyone of her difficulty, not even her mother with whom she generally had an open dialogue. Only three months later, after talking with her philosophy teacher, did the tension ease. The crises kept occurring at every school exam.

When she first came to me, she was in the course of doing another exam; she had done the first part and was preparing for the second.

During our first interview she held her head bent down. While I talked she only occasionally lifted her eyes to look at me and wept abundantly, saying she couldn't control this ceaseless crying and it unnerved her.

Donald Meltzer: We're dealing with an obsessive, repetitive disturbance, even though the patient complains of tension in her back muscles and her difficulty in being with others. One gets the impression her mother has high ambitions for her, perhaps even a too confidential mother–daughter relationship. What is she studying at university?[1]

AM: She is studying at the faculty of humanities.

Chiara is the elder child and has a sister two years younger than her. She talked about her sister during the second session. Her sister had accompanied her to the exam and Chiara was happy with her good results, though 'who knows if I were fatter I might have got a higher mark.' She then talked about her difficulty with food; for two years she had been taking iron pills. Eating gave her no pleasure, she wouldn't chew; her sister, by contrast, enjoyed food and slept well. She always kept an eye on her sister as she ate a lot and Chiara didn't want her to eat more than she did herself. At the dinner table she was always tense, especially if her father was there, whom she described as quick tempered and dissatisfied with his daughters' school performance.

She then brought up her problems at school and thought her success in certain subjects had to do with the teachers' plump physique and her failure at others with their slenderness. At any rate maths and science had been a headache from elementary school: she remembered her trouble with long division; only in her last (fifth) year and with a friend's aid had she mastered it.

DM: This is the second time she mentions receiving help from her friends. The first one was described as an open, extroverted girl friend.

---

1   Meltzer's comments in this chapter were translated from a transcript.

AM: Chiara was filled with tension from the very beginning of the sessions; she'd listen to my words with a schoolgirl's attentiveness, often fearing she had not understood them well. My interpretations were perceived like a judgment that was hard to tolerate. She was keen to control her own words and mine. Negative thoughts which she called her 'aggressive thoughts' were kept away from the sessions; she was afraid I'd be able to see through her and read her thoughts. She felt transparent, as if everyone could see her thoughts, on display, particularly at Mass. Sitting through the entire ritual in the midst of all those people made her suffer intensely.

DM: Didn't she tell you what she thought about during Mass?

AM: No, she only mentioned her uneasiness.

She struggled a long time, fearing she'd lose control if she let herself go and that this would ruin our relationship. She needed to know she could trust me. The negative thoughts emerged from obscurity when there was a change in the setting, about a year after starting the therapy.

DM: How did the setting change?

AM: In September, one of the two sessions was arranged for two hours later.

Chiara was very upset when I changed the session time; I had asked her to come at an awkward time, too close to dinnertime. 'What would I have done with your words?' she asked herself, bewildered. She then started waiting outside, even after her own session, and once she arrived far too early. On that occasion the interpretations regarding her jealousy towards her sister had a strong emotional resonance too.

Her sister was born when she was still very young, she had no words to express her rebellion and felt her sister used up all the milk. 'Your other patients are definitely fatter than you are', she noted.

She experienced me too, like her mother, big and filled with milk, as when she dreamt of me sucking milk with my mouth pressed against hers. Her greed could be linked with her way of studying: she had to learn everything by rote, could leave nothing out; similarly, she had to take down every single word uttered by her teachers. This method filled her with anxiety;

studying and writing really made her suffer. It was possible to relate her first crisis, her writing impediment, to the car accident her mother had in the autumn of her last year at high school. After the accident her mother spent the entire winter in bed and Chiara looked after her personally, recalling that time as a magical period in her life; she was now finally active both at home and school, and joined in discussions with significant and relevant contributions of her own. But her mother's recovery and initial walking on crutches seemed to bring on Chiara's impediment; after that she could not write, especially in Italian classes. She often associated her Italian teacher with her mother.

DM: Obsessive disturbance relates to omnipotent control and separation from parent figures. So this incident with her mother, which kept her mother in bed for a long time, is actually a gift from heaven, a dream of the patient come true.

We can sense that when her mother was expecting her sister, the patient thought her mother was filled with milk, therefore her sister's birth came as a great shock to her. It would be interesting to know how long her mother breast fed; and if this was the case, how the weaning then took place. But knowing these things is not merely for the sake of information or facts, rather as elements emerging from the analytical process.

My impression is that the patient experienced the weaning as a break to allow her mother to fill herself with milk again as Chiara had greedily emptied her mother. Instead she was apparently shocked the moment she saw the result was a young sister, rather than more milk for herself. In addition, Chiara apparently slept in her parents' bed, which enabled her to gain control over them.

My impression is that we're dealing with a patient who is expecting some betrayal and that she has homicidal instincts towards her sister or, I imagine, towards her mother.

AM: We worked on this accident a long while during the first year. In her fantasy, Chiara had to cope with losing her dominant position as mother of the family, since when her mother was ill it was Chiara who ran the house. The identifying and symbiotic bond was once again severed; now her mother was back on her feet resuming her active role, in relation to her daughter and to feeding the family as a whole. By her writing being impeded she became the little girl again, yet guilty of desiring to take everything from her mother, even her position in the household. The fantasy of a dead and wiped-out mother came through the association she made with the shrunken, shrivelled mummy, Roberto, unearthed in an Alpine glacier. Time and again Chiara mentioned her fear of exhausting me with her complaints and negative thoughts, as when in a dream she, while babysitting, looked on passively as her three-month-old sister was flushed down the toilet.

Chiara felt herself to have been ejected before her time, as she was born two months prematurely (had she been born at term, she'd have been in her mother's zodiac sign). Her sister, on the other hand, had remained inside her mother all nine months. At a moment of regression while weeping anxiously, she said she was all alone during her birth, her mother was asleep: she was delivered with a c-section.

DM: We don't know how much she weighed. Was she kept in an incubator?

AM: Yes and I believe she was not breastfed.

DM: This is the story of a patient who has certainly suffered from a precocious emotional deprivation caused by her premature birth and from being kept in the incubator. It's indeed difficult to avoid such a deprivation unless certain signs are noticed as you can read in Romana Negri's beautiful book, due out next year.[2]

Well, this precocious emotional deprivation, which may not derive solely from premature birth but also from a mother's depression, premature separation, a baby's respiratory or intestinal illness – all this leaves in a person's mind and body an unbridgeable gap.

This results for such patients in a very long and repetitive psychoanalytic treatment, being the slow and lengthy achievement of trust. When I talk about the realisation of trust I don't mean acquiring enough trust to become independent, but a slow process of overcoming the tendency to omnipotent control,

---

2   Romana Negri, *The Newborn in the Intensive Care Unit* (2014)

almost a paranoid suspicion. This suspicion is not just pessimism but an expectation of betrayal, which it is feared may occur following an outburst of a homicidal wrath. They are unable to confront delusions, which are seen merely as an anticipation of betrayal. Consequently, they cannot forgive at all and start keeping a catalogue of grievances so long that the psychoanalyst will have difficulty getting over it.

In an analytical situation, it's almost impossible for such patients not to have occasions of resentment which may result in some complaint against the analyst. A slight change in the setting, session hours, even the words spoken, may result in a complaint. They themselves are unable to forgive but keep asking the analyst to be forgiven as they continue to hurt the analyst through their ingratitude and sense of being accused of some guilt. If at any point, in this dismal atmosphere created by the patient, a ray of sunshine should creep in, one wonders 'what has gone wrong?' and whether by chance a certain mental paralysis has occurred, similar to the paralysis of the patient's mother when she had to stay in bed.

In dealing with this obviously unpleasant situation, the analyst does have to hold on to something more fulfilling to maintain a fresh interest in this repetitive process.

How do I deal with this myself in similar situations?

I try to look for a flicker of any undeveloped talent of the patient so as to look for the possibility of developing some positive potential. Otherwise, the learning process remains without a future, as it seems here in the patient's tale of absolutely arid, hopeless school and life experiences. How long has she been with you?

AM: Two and a half years.

DM: How often do you see her?

AM: Twice a week, and recently three times.

Her anorexia became clearer in the context of the first separations in the analysis, denied by both distancing herself physically from the sessions and asserting that she was no longer interested in food, not only in the nourishment of interpretations. By refusing to eat it was she who controlled the separation from food–mother–therapist. Her parents' short trips were associated with the Nazi–fascist alliance; if her mother went away she felt abandoned, but if she was the one who was leaving she was filled with anxiety about being attacked by her mother and me.

After the first year she resumed eating with pleasure; she'd even go to the university canteen. At this time she also started spending more time waiting around after the sessions, especially in the bathroom, getting ready to leave my consulting room.

I perceived she was increasing her control over me and my other patients who followed her sessions; during her own sessions she started touching various objects in the room, looking at the books, but the interpretations failed to limit her intrusiveness. Chiara kept using my study like my younger patients; she literally invaded it and thereby provided me with opportunities to understand what was happening to her.

DM: Did this happen in the course of the second year of therapy?

AM: Yes, in the course of the second year of therapy.

DM: So she passed from controlling to invading you, to being intrusive.

AM: After a dinner she had with her teachers she made critical remarks about her Italian teacher and praised her philosophy teacher. Later on while looking at the flowers on the table, she said they were dirty with pollen, and mentioned that her menstrual period was late. In the following session she came up with the fantasy that her mother would take her to consult a gynaecologist and make her go on the pill to stop her menstrual cycle. She associated her menstruation with anaemia and anorexia.

She dreamed *her mother had a flashy red car which she could drive by remote control and she proudly showed it to a group of men. Just by pressing a button of the remote control in her hand the car would get smaller even though it still remained a wonderful red car.*

DM: At this point we're dealing with the phenomenon of projective identification as a result of her invasion. This projective identification concerns her mother's genitals, and perhaps her father's as well, as we note with the pollen. Its purpose is to control both the sexual act and her mother's menstruation and fertility. She's now passed from external control to internal control of the object; therefore the transference is deeper. At this moment we note the projective identification occurs in relation to the analyst; it's not clear whether being asexual refers to her or to the analyst. She's asking the analyst to be asexual.

AM: She couldn't make up her mind whether to take no sides (remain small and asexual) or assume sexual identity (grow and distinguish herself). She felt relieved when she realised I allowed her to have her menstrual periods.

Before the summer holidays a year ago, she had planned to go away from her family and work in a holiday resort. She had really thought about it but her mother's suggestions made her falter, her initial plan was no longer her own.

DM: Here it happens again with her mother in the same way as with her studies.

It's a lack of trust; if it's true that her mother puts pressure on her, it's because she wants to get rid of her.

AM: At any rate she didn't drop her plan altogether and wouldn't let me help her during the sessions. Interpreting this distancing as a test of her independence, to prove to me and her mother that she had achieved a separation, did not alter her decision; it only meant setting a limit to the planned date of separation to make it more feasible and suitable for her.

DM: I'm reading all this filtered through the way I imagine her first and second year of life: the possessiveness, the confusion with her mother's identity, her expectation of getting back her mother's breast for herself.

AM: The return from the holidays brought in a new era; the separation had been a prelude. Chiara said she felt she'd grown and needed just one session a week. In the first session she related a dream of *an ugly woman, whom she saw to her left and who was charred inside.* (I too am on the patient's left when we sit facing each other during the sessions.) She associated this with a picture of her mother at the seaside with Chiara aged four and her sister aged two. Her mother, she said, looked truly ugly with drooping shoulders and a big protruding belly.

DM: I see it exactly in these terms, as a disappointment.

She feels disillusioned after her return from the summer job, from which she initially expected a lot and which evidently turned out disappointing, as when her mother gave birth to her little sister. In this case there is indeed a rhythm of two years.

AM: After the holidays we were nearly into the second year of therapy and a significantly difficult time awaited both Chiara and me. For several sessions she wouldn't come close to the comfortable easy chair which had become a 'highchair'.

DM: Does she lie on the couch?

AM: Only recently. She felt I didn't want her to do so, I wanted her to remain small. After interpreting her position as a small girl who wanted to keep sitting on the highchair, and since this seemed to frighten her, we decided to meet only once a week for some time. Three weeks later, she complained she was too thin and I remarked this was because she felt little nourished with one session a week. In this period the writing impediment started to recur, which we related to her claim for independence. But her mother decided to pay only for four sessions a month, to which Chiara reacted with fury.

DM: The betrayal!

AM: Her anger soon became physical in the session, as when she went first into the bathroom to defaecate. This made her recall an incident as a child; when her mother was busy with her friends and she needed her attention, she dirtied her pants.

DM: At this point there's a movement, not only a refusal of the analyst and her mother who is seen as defaecating on the analyst, expelling her from her internal world as a charred and dirty figure like faeces. With the magic formula abracadabra she can expel her in this manic and vengeful manner; at the same time she can gain power over the analyst, just as she did previously over her mother when she was ill and bedbound.

Now let's see how the state of the analysis has evolved: it has passed from an initially obsessive state through a deepening of the transference, and has reached a phase of confusion from intrusive identification with the analyst; it has also gone through sexual expectations of owning the analyst and has arrived at a state of disillusion, turning to a manic denigration and expulsion of you and her mother (indistinguishable from one another). So she is now in a manic state of bitterness and triumph over you.

In this manic state of mind patients can be extremely cruel, contemptuous: not only cruel to the analyst and other people but also to themselves, inflicting injuries, burning and cutting themselves.

AM: Resuming sessions twice a week, though, worsened her depressive state. One part of her wanted complete independence while another asked for help. She named her self-sufficient part 'Narcissus', adding she felt that a foreign, unknown body held complete sway over her and thwarted any possible change; therefore Narcissus was her own omnipotent and narcissistic part, the location of her negative thoughts.

Narcissus was the title of a book she'd seen on her mother's bedside table; on its cover there was a picture of a girl with curly blonde hair dressed in nineteenth century clothes; she had thought it might be filled with secrets. The book made her recall a book by Pirandello about the betrayal of a young wife. She later associated betrayal with the words homicide and suicide.

DM: Things are getting worrisome. This book is really a discovery that you have a child of your own: not just patients but a child of your own at home. Your secrets. Does she in fact know anything about your private life, outside of your profession?

AM: I think she knows little about me. Once she came across another patient in my consulting room, just when she was feeling particularly self-conscious, which made her albeit briefly fall into a psychotic crisis; she feared 'Narcissus' would take control of her and I was also quite worried. She then appeared to recuperate, while I had to pay increased attention to her. At the same time, on many occasions one could distinctly perceive her jealousy. During the sessions her constant calls for attention, increasingly more concrete, led me to say that she could not maintain her contact with me outside the therapeutic relationship.

DM: This is a time when patients begin to clamour for physical contact, as evidence of your love for them. At such times the patient succeeds in making you feel that you are killing them.

It isn't just away from the sessions; it's that she cannot manage to find a good relationship with you *in* the sessions; she is mainly being tormented not by the absence of the object but by the *presence* of the object.

I have written about such situations in the book *The Apprehension of Beauty* (1988) in which the emotional impact of the beauty of the object is so intense that the child feels it is being inflicted out of cruelty, unless it is absolutely reciprocated: unless the mother gives evidence that the child is as exquisite to her as she is to the child. This to my mind is the essence of emotional deprivation: when the child's being astonished at the beauty of the mother is not reciprocated by the mother being astonished at the beauty of the child.

This aesthetic impact in the analysis is sometimes visual but of course with a man analyst it is mostly the beauty of the voice that the patient hears as if it were heavenly. In the case of a woman analyst it is much more concretely visual: the patient imagines the beauty of your naked body; little children in this state will beg the therapist to take her clothes off and so on.

The patient's demand for physical contact seems to have the meaning of wanting evidence that their beauty is such that the analyst cannot keep her hands off: just as the patient's hands seem to want to reach out and touch the therapist. But although the craving is for skin to skin contact, fundamentally the impact is visual.

This girl gives the impression of having spent her first year in the parents' bedroom where she had every opportunity of seeing her mother dress and undress.

AM: Indeed she immediately accused me of being cold, distant, and of abandoning her to her sorrows. But my interpretations again failed to effect a change; on the contrary she rejected them then later in the middle of a session asked to sit on 'my lap.'

In the following sessions she tried to claim an exclusive relationship; my interpretations wouldn't help her, to her they were 'poison', as evidenced in a dream she had after asking me to take her in my arms. She was afraid her hostile parts would gain control over her.

AM: At the weekend she made little cuts in her wrists using her father's razor blade.

DM: You had evidence from the period of her intrusiveness of how visual she was – looking into your books but also wanting to touch everything.

AM: At that stage I suggested some pharmaceutical aid and having three sessions a week. We worked on Chiara's difficulty in keeping up a good relation when away from the sessions.

DM: Now about this drug therapy – how did it come about? Was the family getting panicky and wanting a second opinion?

AM: I suggested it, with the patient's agreement.

DM: That probably means you lost your nerve really. It is not surprising given you had very little experience, and you would certainly need the support and encouragement of a more experienced supervisor to be able to tolerate such an onslaught of demands to break your technique. That is essentially what it is: to break your technique as evidence of your love for this patient.

AM: I brought her wrist cuts into relation with an incident which had occurred two years previously. It was in February again at a dinner with her high school girl friends when she had felt judged and excluded, she had made incisions in her wrists. But two and a half years of therapy brought to my mind the age difference between her and her sister. Chiara agreed this could be so, remembered a few sessions previously she had noticed me with a big belly, and burst out into tears, apparently unable to bear being separated.

DM: That's better now. She *sees* you as pregnant. If you imagine a child who sees you as pregnant: on the one hand they see that you are swelling up with milk that you are going to give them, and on the other hand that you are swelling up with a baby that is going to take you away from them, you can see the intensity of the conflict.

AM: Chiara herself in the following session brought up her transitional object: the baby bottle full of milk she'd carry to bed to fall asleep.

DM: This is not a transitional object; this is a *substitute* for the mother – like her period of becoming arrogantly independent of you and demanding to have just one session and so on. The real transitional object is much more of a seducer and a fetishistic object; more sensual. This one is really a substitute.

AM: Once asleep it would slip out of her hands and make her bed stink of milk and urine. This gave us the opportunity to work on the baby bottle with milk interpretation, while the object outside the sessions was emptied to be refilled with corroding pee like her own anger which would renew itself every time she felt abandoned.

Of the many dreams she described I'd like to bring up the first one.

She had already talked about 'Narcissus' and I had already begun to feel a bit anxious about finding myself in a situation anything but simple. Not long after that the dream occurred; she talked about it in the eleventh session, after talking first of another dream. In the dream *Chiara sees a thin fair-haired girl dressed in clothes from the last century. The girl is behind a counter in a square. She gets up abruptly and enters a room with three or four young men; she aims the pistol in her hand at them and kills them, and leaves a white rose on the table. Another young man is by her side and looking amazed he tries to cover up the killing. The girl, undisturbed, goes out into the square again. At one point that girl turns into Chiara herself.*

Chiara, who has straight blonde hair, came to the following session with hair permed and voluminously done up, similar to the picture of the girl on the book cover.

A recent session

DM: So she has been with you two and a half years. So this session is from two weeks ago.

AM: Chiara comes eight minutes late. While waiting for her I think of the previous sessions.

On Tuesday the previous week she had been furious with me and her mother. Her mother had refused to pay for a third session a week, saying she saw little good coming out of psycho-analytical therapy. Chiara thought her mother was not helping her, wasn't giving her enough; while I had made her feel there was something 'wrong' with her by asking her to increase the weekly sessions. Her mother and I showed our selfish greed; her mother did so by withdrawing her financial help and I by asking for more money. Neither of us seemed to satisfy and respond to her needs.

DM: So these are the things you are thinking about while you are waiting for her, during the eight minutes. Not what you were saying to the patient. Sometimes when a patient is late you may review what has been doing on.

AM: The following session (a Friday) she said she feared I might revenge her attacks by counter-attacking her. She imagined seeing me with a beard, like old Freud, with a stern and judging look. The session ended in the corridor and her fantasy of being counter-attacked was calmed. These interpretations also gave Chiara the opportunity to talk about new things she encountered in the outside world and the pleasure she enjoyed in studying and going out with others. I thought the pain she felt during the sessions could relate to her success in experimenting with new things in life, such as being in a group, studying with a girl friend, and suggesting new ways of research to her teachers. Chiara was bewildered by what I said and replied: 'I like hearing such things. Knowing that I'm now taking the initiative and all these nice things happening to me outside are linked with what I feel here with you.' She felt she was now receiving help.

On the Monday session she arrives carrying a very big folder like those that architecture students use. In the corridor she stops and says she smells something, something particular, and says it is 'the smell of therapy'.

DM: Does 'odore' (smell) mean something bad?

AM: No, neutral. Then she said she hadn't made up her mind yet.

DM: She hasn't made up her mind yet. Somebody's been sitting in my chair! It happens in therapy all the time. I have a man patient who really does have a body odour, and the patient who comes after him cannot stand it. It does turn out to mean the smell of her older brother who tyrannised over her; but for a month she really could not bear to come into the room. I am a smoker so didn't smell anything, and finally I asked a colleague to come in who said it did indeed smell in the room.

This kind of sensitivity to smell is very primitive; undoubtedly babies have a very acute sense of smell, like puppies.

AM: When she walks into the study she says she can smell the same perfume here too. She walks to the bunch of freesias on the desk and sniffs at them. It's as if she didn't wish to walk in and sit down. She then says coming here makes her feel 'in therapy'.

Outside she feels fine but here she feels tired, like crying, and she doesn't like that. She then sits across the couch (she has been considering this recently, either sitting across it or lying down on it, depending on her mood). She remembers what we spoke of last Friday and says she'd like to bring beautiful things here to talk about, then turning her head towards me adds 'I love you and you, do you love me?'

DM: Now this has everything in it. Beautiful things. Do you find me as beautiful as I find you. But with a gun to your head!

AM: What if I don't say to her that I love her?

DM: Explain to her the method of psychoanalysis: everybody has to use their own judgement. Otherwise it is 'Do you love me?' 'Yes.' 'Do you really love me?' 'Yes yes …' and so on ad infinitum. This is fundamental to psychoanalysis: nobody can *say* their state of mind, they can only communicate *evidence* of their state of mind, and the other person has to use their judgement.

Participant: It's hard to love such a patient, is this what one ends up communicating then?

DM: It's not true really. To love her as a person is probably impossible; but to love her in a parental way as a suffering baby is quite easy. The expression I used to hear in my childhood was: 'a face that only a mother could love.'

AM: I now remember a Neapolitan saying: 'Every beetle is beautiful to its own mother.' It's true she is a very demanding patient, yet I enjoy being with her.

DM: It's all out in the open now. The secretiveness with which she first presented herself to you has disappeared. Her infantile emotional life is in the open, just as in child analysis. It's the same situation as you'd get with a three-year-old in the playroom. It's very interesting because it is technically challenging. Understanding the material isn't difficult as it is all in the open; but the technical problems of dealing with it and still carrying on with it as an analysis and not a love affair – or a murder – are difficult.

It's the same with any art form. Ultimately the painter isn't interested so much in what he is painting, as in *painting*: paint on canvas is what fascinates him. It's the technical problems of conducting an analysis that makes psychoanalysis so endlessly interesting. To my mind Freud's first stroke of genius was the recognition not only of the existence of the transference, but of the nature of the transference: that the patient wishes you to do something other than analysis with him. This is as true of Kleinian as of Freudian work: regardless of how cooperative the patient may be, there is always pressure on the analyst to *act in* the transference instead of thinking and communicating.

To my mind you have got to the core of this child's emotional deprivation: what I call this aesthetic conflict about whether you are as beautiful inside as she experiences you as being outside. And whether you experience her as a beautiful baby, and see even her urine and faeces as products of the wonders of nature. Never mind that it stinks. It's beautiful that your child produces such healthy-looking faeces.

Another saying about motherhood is: 'She thinks the sun shines out of his little anus.' It's very interesting in baby observation how seldom the observer is allowed to look at the baby's faeces. The nappy is changed so rapidly and precisely that the observer never sees the faeces, but only the expression on the mother's face. Not only the observer: the baby too is watching the mother's face.

Of course in analysis the equivalent of the baby's faeces is dreams of a certain kind, like this one of the girl going and murdering three or four fellows. Such a dream is like a baby with diarrhoea: the mother will either look with disgust at the smelly diarrhoea, or will look worried because her food has not agreed with the baby. There are other dreams that have an impact on the therapist as beautiful faeces that indicate the baby has really digested the milk; because you can see immediately that the patient has digested the previous session. The patient will say, 'You liked that dream!' So just as the baby looks at the mother's face and eyes, the patient in analysis listens for the music of your tone of voice. Not only can you not hide it from the patient, but there is *no need* to hide it from the patient.

I do advise you to explain to the patient about nobody being able to *tell* their state of mind, they can only give evidence of it; she has to use her own judgement about whether you love her or not. You obviously love her sufficiently in spite of the worry, unpleasantness and pain she has caused you. So you are in a good maternal position with her. She is 22 now; as adult to adult she is not a very lovable person; but as parent to child, counter-transference to transference, you obviously love her sufficiently to face up to any scrutiny she makes of your tone of voice.

There are patients that you cannot love. In my experience they are deeply psychopathic patients who have come to analysis with the intention of destroying the analyst – and they sometimes do. Mostly you eventually find out that they actually have criminal activities. I remember one, a rich man who had embezzled a million pounds.

CHAPTER SIX

Hysteria today
(1998)

Hugo Màrquez

We have chosen to present the following case because it offers Dr Meltzer the opportunity to explain his views on hysteria from an array of clinical perspectives while also allowing him to probe into technical difficulties such patients present to the therapist. It is widely accepted that hysterical patients seem to be living out a psychoanalytic text, in particular the theory of the Oedipus complex. As soon as they observe the therapist's interest in them they turn to health matters for shelter, especially if the therapist is a man. Their social success story and triumphant moods are instantly raised like barriers impeding access to the therapist who all too often risks a sharp rebuke such as 'the analyst wants them to fall ill' or 'the analyst finds fault with everything'.

In a similarly resistant transference situation only the concept of pseudo-maturity, as Meltzer notes, can give the analyst enough comfort and strength to persevere and perhaps overcome this technical impasse. Pseudo-maturity is a hypomanic character trait which derives from the hysteria associated with success. Its underlying dynamics consists in projective identification with an internal object (the internal mother) and particularly with an internal part-object (such as the vagina of the internal mother) where the id of the subject dwells, overseeing the sexual traffic and avoiding any possibility of being excluded; this results in repudiating the mother who has been thereby duped and fooled. Very soon the atmosphere of the sessions becomes coloured by tones of triumph, seduction and flirtation, and the therapist will be left wondering how to help the patient to perceive the inauthenticity that results from the constant acting-out and the enfolding social success story. Dr Meltzer stresses the significance of the therapist's gender in transference situations with hysterical patients: the technical difficulties male therapists encounter *vis à vis* manic elements of projective identification, and the difficulties female therapists encounter *vis à vis* claustrophobic elements of the same projective identification. By claustrophobic elements we mean the sort of 'infernal life' which can keep mother and daughter locked together, a trait women therapists are well acquainted with when analysing hysterical patients.

One other technical problem Meltzer emphasises in his supervision of this clinical material is the acting-out situation which wholly conditions the therapeutic relation. During the sessions action replaces communication and therefore it is not the content of the interpretation but the way it is said that is of paramount interest. In projective identification, the patient imposes his mental state on the transference in such an unquestionably domineering manner that everything becomes distorted; the objective is to influence the therapist in such a way that he act out the role assigned to him by the patient's story plot. The therapist soon finds himself caught in a web of circumstances such that he can think of nothing else but complementary countertransference. The patient then consolidates the script imposed through projection, saying: 'You're saying this because you're jealous' or 'You are cold, technical, you don't really care about what's happening to me, just like my mother.' How can one avoid slipping into the role of an excluded third party or of a reticent lover? How interpret a situation without giving the impression that one is saying precisely what is expected?

In such claustrophobic circumstances Meltzer offers two possible helpful remedies for the therapist. The first technical aid consists in describing the transference as the only available resource to allow the patient to come out of projective identification and into contact with their claustrophobic anxiety. In *The Claustrum* (1992) he describes the need to describe to patients in detail the claustrophobic world they inhabit, whose principal characteristic is competitiveness at the highest level for survival, a world where relationships are mostly fake, not sincere. To do this it is necessary to use the material of the patient's daily life, the way he or she experiences the world and its organisation. In addition it is important to describe to the patient what is occurring during the sessions: in the case of Mrs A, the patient about to be described, 'she is like a call girl who comes to the appointment to serve the therapist.'

The second technical aid Meltzer suggests derives from viewing the therapeutic process as an intensely emotional movement aimed at developing immature parts of the personality. Pseudo-mature features generate manic feelings of social success which suffocate tender feelings and suppress depressive values (in the sense of 'depressive position', not 'depressive illness'). Hysterical patients suffer from genital pseudo-maturity which thwarts the development of infantile parts of the personality. For a hysterical patient in projective identification there is no infantile transference, only a stage acting of the Oedipal drama at a genital level; this means it is practically impossible to interpret the drama staged during the transference without the patient believing that the analyst is participating. It is therefore necessary to remove and dissolve the obstacle constituted by the perception 'Daddy's real wife' (in the case of a female patient) or 'Daddy's golden penis' (in the case of a male patient), before pregenital infantile conflicts can start entering the transference. Otherwise the analysis may be broken off or end up being a pseudo-analysis, which thus validates the patient's inauthentic, false self.

The session described below is presented as a paradigm of a claustrophobic atmosphere in the transference and shows the immense technical difficulties the therapist is faced with. Its overriding tone is of the kind 'whatever you say may be used against you.' This is by no means easy on the patient or the analyst. Dr Meltzer's suggestion is truly significant in that it aims to establish a third element, an objective viewpoint from outside this situation that facilitates observation and description of what is going on. The technical advice for finding a way out of the claustrum consists in formulating an accurate and authentic description of the climate in which members of the analytical couple are both immersed. This is the only possible means of real communication left at the analyst's disposal when the projectively identified patient perceives all the analyst's other interpretations as countertransference acts which only strengthen the projective story plot and fail to help the patient observe and reflect about himself.

First consultation with Mrs A

The first contact with Mrs A occurs on the phone early August. She speaks in a very low and serious voice, pronouncing her elaborate words slowly. She asks for an appointment and I give her one in the next week. I'm left thinking she must be a very depressed person. The reason she says she's consulting me are her headaches which don't go away with pills. She is a psychiatrist like myself and works for the health service. She is married to a man 'much older than herself', and has a five year old daughter.

She is wearing elegant and expensive clothes and has a cold, mysterious air. She speaks very slowly, in a low voice, and chooses sophisticated words. Using a highly intellectualised vocabulary she tells me that 'she suffers from a void of affections and is looking for substitutes, fillers.' For a year and a half she has had an emotional obsession with a colleague at her workplace, but all this occurs only on her side as the affair is neither reciprocated nor encouraged by her colleague and she has never talked to him about it. It started when on having to transfer to another work location; she had a passionate dream about him in which they kissed and embraced passionately, and she woke up feeling melancholy and nostalgic. Ever since the dream she has been trying to make it come true in one way or another: she has asked him to be her therapist 'to use the transference already in progress'; she has even suggested he should be her private supervisor. She has never told him directly of her feelings but has only spoken using technical, professional vocabulary. In her view, this affair prevents her 'from falling into a depression'. The previous year in August she called him at work on the phone before the summer holidays; he responded very kindly but talked to her only about a matter which concerns them both professionally, after which she entered a deep depression as this proves he considers her no more than a colleague. She then mentions her 'untimely experiences of death'; at eleven her grandparents died; at seventeen her father; her mother remarried but her mother's new husband died too.

At the end of the interview I tell her I believe her real reason for coming to me is her sentimental attachment. She responds saying it is important for her to understand this situation. After the interview I keep thinking about the confusion between the dream and the real world the patient lives in, the confusion between the present and the past as she phoned me for an appointment on exactly the same day that she had phoned her 'lover' the previous year and whose reaction had highlighted these delusional fantasies.

Donald Meltzer:[1] The patient has made a massive transference between the sentimental situation with her lover and the situation with the therapist. We are now dealing with an immediate process of very intense projective identification. Each time we confront phenomena or situations where one enters or comes out of something, it has to do with projective identification; as in, for instance, claustrophobic perceptions of suffocating or falling down the stairs, or sensations linked with space or spatio-temporal confusions. What Freud says is true, that hysterical symptomology is connected with repression; but a hysterical character, a hysterical personality, is based on projective identification. The hysterical person not only experiences and realises their own fantasies but also experiences and realises those of others, such as those of a parent, a brother. The identification factor in projective identification results in the drama being put on stage and re-experienced again and again.

In a hysterical patient's view, the scope of the therapeutic process consists only in the elimination of the symptoms which

---

1   Meltzer's comments are translated from a transcript.

actually disappear as soon as the transference is established. What then promptly appears and comes to life during the transference is the character structure based on projective identification. Going back to this patient, there are two things worth noting that are relevant to the repetitive nature of the drama: firstly we need to bear in mind that one of the characters of this drama, that is her mother, has lost both her husbands. The second point, as shown in the first part of the session, is the patient's romantic fantasy – that is the drama of two lovers lying together in the same deathbed. This woman's feelings of resentment due to the denial and disillusion caused by her lover are transformed into homicidal desire, according to which he will declare his love for her as he lies dying and the two will die together – a typical nineteenth century fantasy.

Second consultation

The second consultation with Mrs A started with her telling me that last time she felt short of breath while climbing the stairs. Instantly she translates this into intellectualised speech saying it was 'a claustrophobic sensation'. She then starts talking about her falling in love in similar terms to the first session. I remark that I hardly think this can be the only emotion or the only thing she can talk about; I also point out that, for instance, she felt she was suffocating last time. Spurred by these questions, she explains she felt she was suffocating because she thought she'd reached a landing on the stairs, whereas there was none. I then observe that in my view she always keeps another discussion topic ready at hand as a sort of topic-landing, a device for taking a breath and regaining control.

DM: It looks as though the patient comes with a certain programme, an agenda, to control not only herself but also others. This is typical of hysterical patients; they don't just act but engage others in the drama and direct them as it unfolds. One of the difficulties of making observations or interpretations to such patients is finding one's self in a role assigned by the patient; there is no point in saying anything as nothing can surprise or disrupt this mechanism. When the patient says she knows already what the therapist has just said it should be taken to mean she thinks he wants to draw attention to himself. In the patient's drama the role assigned to the therapist is that of an excluded third party, jealous of the love she nurtures for her beloved. It's an instant setup of a triangular relationship.

HM: The patient responds she has only now realised that she can no longer continue this love affair if she wants an analysis. In her view, falling in love was a way of not analysing herself and of escaping from her everyday life. At this point she starts talking about her daily life, of the relationship with her daughter, which suffocated her during the first nine months after giving birth; she could hardly bear her daughter being constantly at her side. She adds her own mother could not help her as she had to look after her second husband, seriously ill at the time.

The meeting scomes to an end and I agree to take her into analysis after giving her a third appointment within ten days to agree on the setting. The patient says she can't come more than once a week due to her work schedule; she also notes that she'd feel guilty if she came after work as this would mean leaving her daughter alone for too long. I inquire how she thinks of solving the matter; she suggests having two sessions on the same afternoon. Obviously I disagree with this and propose two sessions on two separate afternoons until the Christmas holidays (that is for the following three months) and after that three sessions a week. She says she'll let me know her answer by phone; she then phones to say she's having difficulties and will be phoning again later. She does phone to say she'd like to start with two sessions, even if she may not come regularly the first weeks. I reflect thinking this is a rather phobic situation which is impossible to solve outside the therapeutic setting, so I reply by setting the dates of the two weekly sessions. This she accepts.

DM: The patient is actually asking for a non-analysis by phone. Probably she likes the phone and enjoys using it as teenagers do. A telephone enables an internal communication to be heard by someone else. The claustrophobic person asks the outside person for help on the phone; this mechanism can also involve other personality traits, such as an infantile aspect asking for help from another more mature part on the outside. Speaking on the phone in adolescence can at times have a dream-like quality, partly because while talking on the phone we don't really know what's happening at the other end of the line; it isn't a real contact. A state of suspense exists, and a lack of trust which may come to life within the transference, as the patient cannot view the analyst's sitting position. Some patients manage to control the analyst in minute detail: they hear him breathe, feel when he looks at his watch and so on. Many patients need to receive constant proof that they are receiving attention and that there's contact between the analyst and themselves.

Some significant relationships

Mrs A describes her mother as 'always commanding and harsh'; she worked with her husband abroad and was almost always away from home, which is why she attended a religious boarding school run by nuns, from kindergarten to high school.

DM: The patient evokes the impression of having been neglected as a child.

HM: Her father she describes as 'a fascinating man who adored me and fulfilled all my wishes; he'd come to visit me from abroad at boarding school, I'd go out to dinner or to the cinema with him and I enjoyed having people think I was his partner. He'd buy me beautiful clothes, and used to say I had aristocratic blood and would need to choose a man with extra care; he was jealous of me.' Her adored father died of blood cancer when the patient was seventeen. She states she'd known it in a dream even before receiving the news of his death. She was by his side throughout his illness, 'and at the end he was like a saint, a God'.

DM: It's as if such dreams are for the patient not simply dreams but a sort of communication enabling her to contact her father, a sort of religious communication. There is a feeling that this hysterical child nurtured the fancy of being daddy's little wife, a fantasy that can be viewed as projective identification in the sense of being as if she had sexual relations with him, as if she'd received her father's penis by staying inside her mother. The telephone communication holds the meaning of communication between two different places. This type of dream also holds the meaning of communication between two different places – between the present moment and the afterlife. In this special relationship between her and her father, the mother is apparently being presented as the one who doesn't know what's going on, a stupid mother, unaware of things.

HM: Her husband is seventeen years her senior. 'Perhaps I married him to provide my mother with a husband rather than myself.' The patient comes from a social and economic class above her husband's; even in psychological terms he's described as the 'weaker one'; she has driven him out of their bedroom and has had no sexual relations with him for years.

DM: A sadistic punishment as he is the husband-father she doesn't wish to have.

HM: When she became pregnant she broke off the psychotherapy she had begun a short time before. She talks of her daughter mostly to express her feelings of inadequacy and guilt for not finding enough time to be with her; her mother and her husband actually look after her daughter.

DM: Patients with a negative identification with the same-sex parent take the conscious decision to behave completely differently towards their own children once they themselves become a parent; what actually happens is that eventually they almost inevitably repeat the very mistakes they've criticised their parents for. Conscious negative identification is not as powerful as unconscious positive identification; hence the drama of their own childhood repeats itself and we suspect that between her own husband and the daughter the same sort of relationship is being played out as the patient felt she herself had with her own father. In hysterical patients we repeatedly come across the drama of feeling excluded while secret relations are taking place somewhere else. Treating hysterical patients is extremely difficult; the symptoms disappear relatively quickly when the transference sets in, but the illness establishes itself during the transference through the deployment of the same characteristics; this is what poses the major difficulty to their treatment. The history of their therapy is characterised by continually going into and coming out of therapy. Owning the problem of a character based on projective identification means also acknowledging the fact that the adult part of the personality is only pseudo-mature.

Such patients' relationships are only superficially problem-free; real difficulties arise in intimate relationships. Social adaptation is of manic type in that they find satisfaction in the success their pseudo-maturity affords them. Therefore the principal goal of the analysis is to mobilise the other side of projective identification, which is claustrophobic anxiety. Such patients are able to assume a cooperative and eager approach to analysis, but it is not sincere. As a matter of fact, what happens is a continual enactment hidden in the transference, where a triangular relation is imposed. If one looked back into the history of the preceding therapy or therapies the patient may have had, one would undoubtedly see they were all broken off with some excuse; in this way it is always the analyst who is the abandoned one. The case of Dora is a typical example of a failure in treating a hysterical patient.

The real difficulty in therapy is to succeed in mobilising the claustrophobic anxiety so it emerges in the transference. This can be achieved by interpreting the continual acting-in during the transference in seemingly cooperative situations which, however, are in point of fact only a pseudo-cooperation. These patients do not leave analysis because they feel claustrophobically trapped, but rather because they feel or believe they've succeeded in manipulating the therapist, imposing on him a countertransference reaction; or else they believe the analyst has fallen in love with them, or they themselves are jealous as the analyst has not fallen in love with them. In general, one could say it's much better if the analyst is of the same sex as the patient. It's easier for a hysterical patient to have a female analyst succeed in mobilising the persecutory claustrophobic anxiety, which is her real problem.

It's very important to understand the nature of the difficulty in analysing a hysterical personality because in the course of any psychoanalytical process we come to the Oedipus complex and this must be analysed. With such patients one cannot analyse the pregenital Oedipal complex without drawing the patient out of projective identification; everything seems genital until the analyst achieves this. Only then, for the first time, will the pregenital complex become accessible. The techniques for getting the patient out of projective identification are mainly those of not enacting the countertransference and of describing in detail to the patient what is happening here and now: the claustrophobic world the patient actually lives in. The first stages of analysis – which for such patients may continue for a year or two – are wholly dominated by this acting-out in the transference. There is no maternal transference until the patient is taken out of projective identification.

Projective identification always generates two types of phenomena: 1) a projective claustrophobia of being enclosed, held inside; 2) a projective aspect of a manic nature. Male hysterical patients usually identify with the penis of the internal father. One way to weaken the identification enforced by the pseudo-mature part of personality is to accurately note and explore the fraudulence: not only what the patients themselves feel to be fraudulent but also the suspicion that others view them as fraudulent. Noting and describing the claustrophobic world they inhabit brings them into contact with claustrophobic anxiety. The principal feature of this claustrophobic world is intense competition for survival: it's a world where relationships are mostly hypocritical and insincere.

In order to describe the claustrophobic world, one has to use the material brought by the patient themselves about their work or daily life, in order to show how they experience the world and its organisation. The external world can naturally evoke all sorts of feelings: feelings of affection, love, murderousness – it all depends on the kind of patient. For instance, hypomanic patients evoke a world of frivolous things, whereas more paranoid patients see a world full of suspicion. For a hysterical patient in projective identification there is no infantile transference; what exists instead is a staged genital Oedipal drama in which the patient believes that the analyst is taking part in the role projectively assigned to him.

Some significant biographical information

At the age of thirteen or fourteen the patient started suffering from acute headache. Simultaneously another symptom occurs in her legs: she's no longer able to stand on her feet, often falls down though without fainting; for this reason, at the boarding school, she needs to be taken in someone else's arms to go down to classes and up to the halls of residence.

DM: The symptoms of hysteria usually start to appear in puberty.

HM: In her pre-adolescent years (that is before the age of thirteen or so), she says she was being 'disobedient' at school: 'I'd make demands as a representative of the entire group of girls; I refused to go to Mass; I'd stand up and speak out on behalf of others. Little by little though they chained me down until I stopped joining in with the rest of the class in the last year of secondary school.' She was put under the assistance of a tutor who eventually won over her.

DM: This is how the patient herself describes the claustrophobic way in which she experiences the world; it is the world where her father would come to rescue her, whereas her mother-educator would enslave her in it and persecute her. It's a highly political world of power struggle: between the old and the young, the rich and the poor. In puberty and adolescence such a struggle is a struggle for sexual freedom in conflict with parents. In spatial terms, this power struggle occurs in the mother's body, in the genital space, but moves to the rectum as tyrannical and sadomasochistic perversions begin to develop.

The analytical situation during the first year

There were a series of difficulties regarding the setting in the analytical situation. Mrs A was against having the necessary number of sessions to achieve a more or less functional analytical process. She couldn't come twice weekly during the first three months of analysis and couldn't begin a three sessions a week schedule during the first year. I had to keep up the continuity when she failed to do so and risked breaking off the process several times. In my view stopping this analysis would have been harmful after she had previously abandoned two previous therapies. The patient always accused me of not understanding her reasons, and of being more interested in her technical motivations and explanations rather than herself as a person. She often felt guilty for not dedicating enough time to her daughter. Her mother and her husband, as she put it, 'opposed her analysis all the time.' The true and sincere explanation for not increasing the weekly sessions was finally accepted by the patient when she said she would act in the same way when a relationship started weighing down on her. This is how she felt during the first analysis where the analyst 'pushed her to deepen the relationship' without understanding that 'he wouldn't achieve this as she preferred to go only up to a certain point, particularly if the analyst is a man.' This is now also what happens with her mother and her daughter, though. The first thought that crosses her mind when she begins a relationship is: 'What if this person should die?'

As for the topics discussed, the first year of analysis soon went well beyond the patient's imaginary love life to concentrate on the transference situation. The analytical relationship then began wavering between an idyllic state and a threatening and dangerous one, between accusations of insensitivity, indifference towards the analyst, and strong attempts to control him. Before the summer holiday break such persecutory feelings increased remarkably, with dreams of children's heads with eyes staring at the patient wherever she was – in the toilet, on the car bonnet and so on.

After the summer holidays the patient did not come back immediately but called to say she'd be away one more week. When she eventually did come back, she said if she had come sooner all the desire to return which had obsessed her when away from therapy would have ceased to exist. Of her holidays she recalled a sentence with absolutely no meaning from a dream: 'A deadly chaos is investing the traffic of index fingers.' She could make no associations to this, while I thought to myself it had to relate to masturbation. After the summer holidays she went back to talk about her imaginary sentimental relations, saying she nurtured no 'sublime feelings' towards me as she still does towards the object of her desire. She brought no other dreams.

Some dreams from the first year of analysis

This is a dream Mrs A had after the second consultation, when she failed to make up her mind whether she should start analysis or not: *You were there* [the analyst] *and Fabio* [her lover], *but the two faces blur and overlap and form a third person sitting in a room much cosier than this one and talking to me in a gentle, warm voice as I like to be talked to. The person was saying I'd be able to make my decision and that I had to say clearly if I wanted to go into analysis or not.*

She observes that it was a decisive dream as she 'decided the following day to take on the pain that analysis entails.'

DM: With the dream she also illustrates the quality of the mental state she lives in: not cosy.

HM: A dream she had after the first session of the analysis: *I dreamt I was in labour, giving birth to a girl; I held her in my arms. There were my husband, my existing child, very jealous, and my mother, as always intrusive, telling me what to do and what not to do.*

DM: There are the people who form part of the drama.

DM: Another dream: *I dreamt of giving birth to five children; my mother was there and said it was a whim of mine to have all those five children.*

DM: Masturbation.

HM: In the next dream: *You* [the analyst] *and I were together in my mother's car; the car wasn't moving, the seats were reclined, and we were sitting; I see an erect penis but don't know if it was yours. You push something in my mouth with your hands; you make a cup with the palm of your hand, filled with my menstrual blood, you make me drink it. The car is stained all over. Then you open the car door and walk out; I'm left worrying as it's my mother's car, I want to wash off the stains but can't find the keys, I'm distraught. I cover the rear seat with a piece of cardboard and go home. My mother comes with a brown cat which can be blown up like a* *balloon through its tail; my mother shows me how to do it but I say this could harm the cat; so my mother puts it in my arms, I hold it tenderly and wonder how to hold it without making my mother get angry.*

Her associations to this dream were that when having sex she used to think of her mother and could go no further. She would feel guilty because she was a widow whereas she herself could have sex and this felt like spiting her so she gave up sexuality. In the summer by the sea her daughter sleeps with her mother and she with her husband. Her mother asks her to make the same sleeping arrangements as at home, where she doesn't sleep with her husband anyway; at home her daughter sleeps in the same bed as she does; this all started when the child was little and couldn't fall asleep, so to avoid a sleepless night she took her into her own bed.

Mrs A explains that as a child she would first go to bed with her father and then slip into her own little bed, which had brown sides, when she heard her mother's footsteps; her father also pretended to be asleep. Later when she was around thirteen or fourteen she was often at home together with her father, who'd come from abroad to visit her at the boarding school and she would sleep with him in the king-size bed on her mother's side. When he fell ill he left the king-size bed to sleep in her own bed, and she went to bed with my mother. She went back to sleep in her own bed after he died.

DM: Going back to Dora, her oral symptoms clearly suggest the fantasy that Mr K stands for the father's penis and Mrs K is sucking the penis; all this takes place inside the maternal vagina. This fantasy is the pregenital background conflict which in hysteria appears as if it were genital. This pregenital background is manifest in the confusion between the penis and the nipple, consequently the mouth is mistaken for the vagina and the same goes for the hand. The dream where she is giving birth to five children is a fantasy of the five fingers of the masturbating hand transformed into five newborn babies.

The problem the analyst eventually finds himself facing, when he makes interpretations to this patient, is that of being able to talk without the patient's viewing it as the result of their influence over the analyst who has merely assumed the role assigned to him in the predominant fantasy of the transference.

A typical session

This is a typical session from a year and two months after the beginning of the analysis. The patient says she is feeling confused, pulled in all directions, in conflict and deeply anxious; she has similar feelings during the sessions too. She'd like to talk to me but fears saying ordinary or silly things; my being there conditions her, so she ends up talking only about the things she thinks I'd accept.

DM: It's not clear whether she's complaining or being seductive; she's hesitating between being plaintive and compliant.

HM: She continues saying she's therefore so uneasy and confused that she would like to contact another therapist in order to be able to tell him the things she can't say to me; she knows it would be a mistake and finally withdraws into herself.

DM: It's quite strange that a patient at this point in analysis should consider consulting another therapist, so one must believe it's serious when she says it. It's difficult to say something when a session begins in this way, for whatever one says will be experienced as a reaction such as: 'Make up your mind. You either stay with me or go away.'

HM: She then says she no longer has a headache but knows that when she does have it, whether it gets worse or not depends on the analysis.

DM: The analyst is responsible for her mental state; it's the analyst's qualities which cause or alleviate her mental state.

HM: She then continues saying she's afraid of making a bad impression, of saying negative things about herself. She thinks she's not free enough to talk as I'm not a stranger to her; every time she's about to say something, something I myself say impresses her, leaving her blocked, preventing her from talking further.

DM: Whatever the analyst may say is taken either as a reassurance or denial because her entire mental state, her entire being depends on the analyst. It's important to describe to her what is actually happening during the sessions: that she experiences the analyst as a particular object in a particular place whose features are the result of transferring her mental state onto a current situation. For instance, she might say she's feeling like the analyst's slave and that whatever she thinks or says is done to please him but she doesn't know how to. The patient is experiencing a sort of persecutory slave–master relationship, with its masochistic connotations. It's necessary to describe to her the actual state of things: that in the session she is feeling and behaving like a slave who is trying to gratify, satisfy whatever wish of her master. Or else one can also tell her that she is feeling like a sort of call-girl who comes to the appointment to serve her client, the analyst.

HM: The patient says she'd like to probe further and come three times a week, but that she's afraid of this; the more the analyst goes deeper, the less she can talk; she's afraid of disappointing, of harming or of putting heavy, unrealisable demands on the analyst ...

DM: Just like with her lover with whom she could not speak frankly and normally. From the very beginning the patient has mistaken the analyst as her lover, perceiving him as superior to herself and feeling full of sexual desire as a subservient slave towards her master; whereas she feels no desire for her husband whom she thinks of as her inferior. The notions of superiority and inferiority which colour the world the patient lives in are hierarchic social-economic concepts, characteristic of the claustrophobic world. The patient is gradually denigrating her lover in relation to the analyst; she's continually lowering him to the point of making him kiss her genitals; for the patient this equals humiliation, for she felt she was in a position where she had to suck his penis to give him satisfaction and now she's trying to reverse the situation with him. It's a context of oral sexuality.

HM: She then says that what she hates most in her relationship with her husband is feeling superior to him, whereas with Fabio it is the other way. I comment that perhaps she can't talk to me as she's afraid I may disappoint her. She says no, it's she who is afraid of disappointing me: adding she intuitively knew I'd intervene as I interrupt her every time she begins to talk about Fabio.

DM: She forces the analyst to be particularly attentive as to when to intervene, as she interprets his words as exhibitionism, or else as an expression of his jealousy of her relationship with Fabio. For the patient whatever the analyst says during the session is acting out his countertransference as she sees it; she's not so much concerned with the content of the analyst's comments as with the action implicit in talking. She observes his behaviour, pays attention to his tone of voice, rather than to what he interprets.

HM: She says she feels differently about her lover now from what she used to and that this change is the fruit of the analysis; she no longer idealises her lover she says but recognises his limits; and she no longer feels attraction or desire towards him but only profound rage for wasting so much love on nothing.

DM: The patient is now trying to reassure the jealous analyst; she doesn't love Fabio but him. But implicitly she is also threatening the analyst: beware, don't disappoint me because what has happened to Fabio may happen to you too! Such a way of treating the analyst implies that she conceives analysis as a situation in which people threaten, blackmail and control one another; they impose themselves on one another, or give in to one another. She doesn't see analysis as a place for a reciprocal sincere relationship of esteem, trust, and meaningfulness. If the analyst slipped into the patient's mentality he'd also begin to feel tense, afraid of speaking his mind to the point of no longer being able to speak, as happened to her with respect to the analyst. Thus the patient would reduce the analyst to silence.

The same situation can occur between couples who can no longer talk to one another from fear of being inferior to the other, of disappointing the other, of not being up to the mark. I'd like to emphasise strongly that there's a big difference between communication and action: that in the claustrophobic world there is no communication but only threatening and manipulation and so on. Such a state in an analysis is a mutually persecutory one. This will become progressively clearer in the patient's dreams; as the persecution gradually increases, the times of separation (weekend, breaks etc) become ever more filled with acting-out.

HM: She states she allows herself to be attracted by the wrong people; neither Fabio nor her mother or husband have empathised with her, understood or treated her with respect. This might have to do with the fact that she perhaps would have enjoyed seeing them resemble herself just a little! She also adds her husband is tormenting her as he refuses to meet her mother and there's no way to reach a compromise. She has suggested undertaking a couple therapy, but he replied it's she who needs the therapy because it's her mother's fault. In the meantime, when she's out at her sessions, he profits from her absence to strengthen his relationship with their daughter. If they were to separate one day, he'd walk off with their daughter. She is filled with immense rage but restrains herself and afterwards she's got a headache and is about to faint. She can hardly make her way to the door.

DM: The patient is asking the analyst to agree with her and to regard her as a woman full of excellent qualities whereas it's the bad people who give her a headache. She's viewing the analyst as her equal, which is why she's asking him to see eye to eye with her. She lives in a world of agreements, alliances, deals and compliance instead of sincere friendships. It's a world in which people ally with one another because they have common foes against whom they should form a bond; consequently, she wants the analyst to agree with her that her husband is their common enemy. If the analyst actually were to do so, she'd secure herself an ally; but this would mean abandoning his analytical position by shifting onto the patient's side, as her father used to do.

HM: I told her that as much as she tries, despite all the attempts she feels she's making, she feels none of her relationships match up to the one with her father.

DM: One of the most difficult and most risky features with such patients who idealise a parent is to tell them anything they might regard as criticism of their adored daddy. It is, however, important to describe to her the idealised nature of her relationship with her father and how she's attempting to repeat the same situation with the analyst; but care is also needed not to describe these qualities as her father's real character traits but as how the patient herself perceives and experiences them. She's united in alliance with her father against her mother. You need to be very careful because if the patient detects criticism of her father she'll feel the analyst is being jealous of her relationship with her father, so the analyst could fall from the height where she has placed him and she would feel free to break off the analysis.

In fact, the patient places her father in a very negative light, like a person with whom she has a sexual relationship behind her mother's back; but this needs to be listened to as the manner in which the patient experiences her relationship with her father, not as her father's actual behaviour. I'd suggest you should not talk with her about her father until she's come out of projective identification, after which she'll be able to talk with the analyst more frankly and with less confusion.

HM: To my interpretation she responds she'll try to remember what I've told her because this might open up her mind later on, but now she's closed it and has forgotten it. She asks me to repeat it. She asks if this means that she was in love with her father.

CHAPTER SEVEN

An egocentric adolescent
(1998)

Mauro Rossetti

At the beginning of September 1991 I get a phone call from a young man's father. A neurologist acquaintance has told him to contact me and he is asking me to take him into therapy. I note some haste in his request, the father wishes me to start very soon. He also adds the boy is quite big and mature enough to come to me on his own, which makes me conclude that he and his wife do not intend to speak directly with me.

I then ask the young boy to contact me, which he does the following day. We set an appointment. Enrico arrives punctually. He is tall and ugly as any adolescent can be while moving out of puberty into adolescence. But he has gentle, mild manners. All in all he is an agreeable boy.

He tells me his problems started when he was sixteen. He fell madly in love with a girl in his class and ever since can't help thinking of her night and day. His school performance deteriorated, he can't sleep and has become isolated from others. 'Before that I was fanatical about my studies which used to be my only interest in life. When I started high school, I studied less and less and now feel under growing pressure. Sometimes

I throw up before leaving for school.' At night he'd often run to the window at the sound of the passing waterbus, hoping to get a glimpse of Maria, the object of his infatuation; and often he even happened to 'see her' but later realised it couldn't have been her (as it was 4 or 5 in the morning!).

What is particularly significant in all this is that Enrico has in actual fact never genuinely approached Maria. Through their common friends he sent word of his interest in her, and through the same channel he was told she had no interest whatsoever in him. The two never spoke of it, just chatted about general things and always in the company of others. In the sessions Enrico often talks about Maria and his 'memories'; when I inquire about these I discover that these are his fantasy story which is now being treated as real and authentic. Enrico knows these things have never existed, but then contradicts himself, saying he lives 'in the past.' Enrico says: 'When I started university the separation I felt was painful. Maria started university too but she refused to see me.' (Maria is studying for a degree in medicine.)

Enrico's father works as an engineer in a company, has undergone a deep depression and neurological therapy. His mother, a housewife, has also had some medication, but he doesn't remember the details. He has a younger sister in her last year at high school. She has a boyfriend and a good group of friends. Enrico doesn't speak much about her, as he doesn't about the rest of his family.

When Enrico's parents grew aware of his state, they decided a change of air would do him good. They sent him to live in a different town with his grandparents and he was enrolled in a new school. Enrico lived with his grandparents for only a year, a period he described full of immense emotional conflict; he felt lonely, out of place, away from his love, forced to live with two elderly persons he couldn't understand, and to socialise with people of his age with whom he had nothing in common. He came back to Venice and with difficulty managed to conclude his studies. He is now in his second year studying for a degree in engineering, but so far has not sat a single exam.

First meetings

During our first interview I felt on the one hand interested in this young man who talks pleasingly and with such concern about his problems; but on the other hand I also feel some distortion, something falsified in all this: starting with the way the father phoned to arrange the first meeting. Towards the end of the consultation Enrico tells me he must sit a university exam to postpone conscription. Inconsistently, he also boasts that he is studying for two or three subjects at the same time, one of which is particularly important, and believes he can pass them all.

Now I believe I can grasp the family's haste, his father's equivocal phone call and the young man's opaqueness with me. I go over in brief what he has been telling me and confirm that he can undertake therapy (noting his introspective capacities), but that in order to help him I require certain conditions which guarantee continuity and stability in our relationship. The problem of military service unfortunately does not provide the necessary security and I have no magical power to achieve in a short time what he himself hasn't done in two years. So I ask him to deal with that question first: either he enters the military service or he sits the university exams. Once this is settled we can start therapy. I suggest he should abandon his grandiose plans, such as studying for a number of subjects in a short time, and concentrate on one light-weight exam if he wants to avoid conscription. I then say good-bye and suggest he keep in touch and tell me how he's getting along. Enrico leaves in the same courteous and amiable manner as he appeared at the beginning of the interview, with no apparent sign of frustration.

The following day his father phones and I tell him what I've told his son.

Nearly a month afterwards Enrico rings to tell me he's tried to follow my advice but he's now facing serious difficulties. I believe his need for help is genuine and give him an appointment.

In the course of this second interview I suggest having a series of sessions until December exclusively to come to grips with the current problems; after that we should decide if and how we should go on.

Enrico comes promptly to these sessions, passes an exam (with the lowest possible mark). In January we start the analysis with three sessions a week. Now we're meeting four times weekly.

I've always had the impression I made a mistake with his parents who are like phantoms to me. I believe I'd be much more tranquil today if I had met them for an interview first; I believe I've missed a chance and that now it's too late.

Donald Meltzer: In therapy with such young men it's always better not to see the parents. Otherwise there's the risk of becoming their agent and then much time is needed to overcome this obstacle. It's a little as if the parents were employing you to do what they themselves hadn't succeeded in doing.

MR: Wouldn't it have been the same even if I had actually met them?

DM: With fourteen to fifteen-year-old adolescents it can be helpful to also meet their parents; after sixteen it's better to see the teenagers on their own, otherwise there's the risk of being regarded as the parents' agent, parents' representative.

MR: I think his parents are like phantoms to me because they send their son to have therapy with someone they don't know, however well one of their acquaintances may have spoken about me; they tend to minimise their son's problems, spend money, and he doesn't even do his exams, nothing!

DM: The parents of adolescents must deal with the question of losing their influence, so it can happen that they're more than happy to delegate their own responsibility. They feel whenever they try to intervene they succeed in nothing but provoking negative reactions from their son.

One other drawback in meeting the parents is that this may, in analysis, affect the encounter with internal parents who can be very different from the real ones.

Progression of the therapy: autumn and winter 1991

One day Enrico came to a session and said: 'Today I've been at university feeling completely lost, with an intense urge to escape, it was like going back to the "crime scene". People I met by chance made me feel ill at ease. Though I mostly knew them well, I felt they were judging me.'

One of the major problems I've had with Enrico in therapy is the heavy drowsiness he induces in me. The other matter regards his ceaseless talk: the moment he lies down on the couch he starts talking without stopping to the very end of the session. If I intervene, Enrico keeps politely silent until I stop and then he resumes his talk. Whether I talk or not doesn't seem to have any relevance for him. In the following session, though, he refers to what I said the previous time and what he's thought about between the sessions.

DM: Now you can understand why Maria does not want to see him: because he is boring! He's affected by a sort of obsessive boredom, he is an obsessive person. Were he a more attractive young man there'd naturally have been different repercussions; but he's evidently boring, shallow and not very good-looking. Often it happens that young men who have been doing well in latency, bent on their studies, working hard to fulfil their ambitions and expectations (perhaps not really their own but those of their parents'), transfer their obsession in puberty when they meet someone of the opposite sex who then becomes the object of obsession. Such young men may have had good results at school during latency because of their solid memory, and their capacity to respond adequately and recount facts, though all without any genuine imaginative power of their own. At the same time they fall in love and take a quasi-obsessive interest in the boy or girl. They are entrapped in an obsessive, monotonous circle whose object remains the chosen person; then they nurture fantasies of an often non-existing relationship which tends to take the place of reality. If the fantasy is transformed into a real social action, its results are wild, delirious, as everything is based on a hypothetical relationship which in fact doesn't exist.

A young man like Enrico, once immersed in his fantasies, is likely to take a bunch of flowers to the girl of his desires with the same naturalness as a husband would to his wife to celebrate their wedding anniversary; but instead of evoking interest, excitement or pleasure, he only ends up causing discomfiture. It's a rather crazy, out of place gesture.

Participant: What's the difference between this sort of obsession and erotic-manic delirium? Between this patient and Nathaniel and Olympia's doll by Hoffmann which Freud describes in 'The Uncanny'?

DM: This young man is in his latency, his eroticism is not strong yet; he may be masturbating a little but what he mainly does is ruminate. Naturally if he were to meet a similar partner they'd fall in love and make what I myself describe 'a doll's-house couple'. Such a couple could well get married, have children, and do the usual things (work and so on), but in solitude, with few friends, staying inside their house of dolls where the game can be kept up. But it seems to me that Maria isn't that sort!

Participant: Doesn't that sort of ruminating that he has about Maria and his love relationship also exist with the analyst, from the first sessions? For instance, the way he goes back to what the therapist has said in the previous session, precisely as though he'd ruminated over his words before absorbing them.

DM: With this information alone it's too soon to tell the role and function the analyst occupies in his mind. Without doubt, though, Enrico is dealing with certain problems his parents hadn't known how to solve for him, and he may be waiting for the analyst's intervention to solve them.

MR: I'll now tell you the first full dream he talked about in a session. Enrico was *in a big house with lounges and enormous rooms; there were other people, and they were all terrorised by a giant, a monster. They had time to hide because it would come punctually at set times. At such a time he would hide in a bed or under it, or behind a door. People would wonder anxiously how they could avoid the monster. It was very tall and so its face was not visible.*

DM: It's rather like the story of the mouse that tries to sort out what to do with the cat. At a certain point the mice decide to hang a bell around the cat's neck in order to hear its approach; but the real question is how to tie the bell around the cat's neck!

This dream certainly has to do with the transference and what the analyst signifies in the patient's life. Each time the therapist opens his mouth to speak it's as if he roared to swallow him. At this point the patient is terrorised by his therapist, perhaps because you are the cat and he is the mouse.

However, let me underline a positive thing in this dream: Enrico is not alone against the terrible monster, he's in the company of other mice that together make up a congregation of scared mice. His friends are asexual relations: a brigade of mice! In fact Enrico doesn't know how to hide, whether on top or under the bed or behind the door.

MR: The previous day Enrico had said he considered himself an eternal loser, of little significance for others and not at all attractive. His talk with others in the dream makes me think of his ceaseless chatter during the sessions which leaves no room for anything else. His association to the dream was: 'I thought it was my other self which stopped and blocked me.'

I interpreted the dream as on the one hand he feels like a monster with all the rage inside him, on the other he perceives me as a monster: before me he's like a defenceless child looking for shelter in daddy's and mummy's bed.

Next session, the following day, he says: 'I thought a lot about your interpretation yesterday. But I'm convinced the dream represents my other self …' and so on.

DM: Enrico doesn't regard himself much as a monster and when the therapist offers ideas which transform him into one, he questions the latter's interpretation. He wants to challenge him but doesn't know what to substitute him with. He is the monster, a part of himself is monstrous, and the monster's features are as follows: He doesn't study, doesn't do sports, doesn't succeed in anything. There's nothing actually monstrous about him, but what he certainly wishes to do is to question what he the therapist says and refute his ideas.

MR: Enrico continues: 'Many ideas rush into my head but I do nothing; I've got ideas about my studies, sports, TV, but don't know what I feel and end up not stopping at one single thought.'

I hint at the confusion he may be feeling mentally. He says 'Yes, there's a black-out, I'm excited, I feel ideas come up and go down but all in vain. I don't know what to do. It's like a circle of ideas that keep going round, one rubbing out the other, always the same things' (he sounds plaintive but not desperate.)

DM: This is a clear description of the ruminating process which keeps going round in circles.

MR: I feel confused too now as he talks without stopping in his monotone. At one point as he's describing what he does in the morning and at home, he says: 'Could it be fear of hollowness? The search for pleasure as comfort and serenity?'

I try to understand if he's referring to masturbation without mentioning it, but his talk changes to what he imagines is happening in sports events and how he enjoys this fantasy. I even thought he might be desperate about compulsive masturbation but couldn't find a way to open up that subject; I doubted if it would be of any use to say so.

As I try to fight against the torpor induced by his incessant talk, I tell him he's worried as he's once again facing fragmented thoughts, to which he replies by cutting me short: 'No! They are crumbs of thoughts!'

DM: 'They are not fragments but crumbs': it's negativism. He's trying to counter the therapist in an undefined, vague way.

Participant: Does 'no' mean fear of falling into excessive dependence?

DM: I think I note a lot of anger against people who know what to do where he doesn't and who try to teach him; he has little trust in the people who take on a paternal role, who try to teach him something to help him become a more virile man; he thinks they're making fun of him, they're humiliating him. It's as if he were a small baby attracted by his mother but aware of the father between himself and his mother. A small baby fighting his father to the last drop of blood to get his mother, knowing full well his father won't help him at all and he'll always remain a rival to fight against.

MR: At the end of that session Enrico says: 'I recalled high school and my teachers. I remembered the philosophy teacher with a lot of anger.' As he says this I feel he pulls himself together, he composes himself in however paranoid or melancholic a state; I think he sees me as like his philosophy teacher who failed to understand him, but I accept this feeling because at the moment there isn't much I can do to change it.

The following session Enrico starts by saying he'd like to be understood and to establish a new kind of dialogue. He talks of imagining a conversation with that teacher to tell him who he really is and to ask him what he didn't understand in class. He continues saying that later at home he imagined a volleyball game which had never existed. 'Certain monologues end up being a record.'

I suggest, perhaps in order not to hear the silence and feel the solitude.

He says: 'Yes, when this imaginary sports event started my mother and my sister were at home, but I was alone in my room and could not take that off the record. I kept going into rooms and didn't want to stay in a single one. I don't think I can stop myself feeling hollow: but I can't fill the space up either with my mother, my sister, the radio or the TV. Sometimes I keep the radio on all the day. Sometimes I write something about fear, solitude, silence. Sometimes I feel like a monster. I've written my last will over and over again, sometimes I feel like I can't breathe.'

DM: As a matter of fact this is recycling, a highly painful and moving description of his suffering: 'alone in my room,' 'so much that he couldn't take off the record,' 'can't defend myself against solitude'. When he mentions his last will he must really be desperate: poor fellow. This certainly has to do with his sister's birth and his feeling that she had taken his mother away from him. When Enrico mentions to his sleepless nights and the waterbus he sees pass at 4 or 5 am, he is actually referring to his mother who'd get up to feed the newborn baby she'd take in her arms and carry from one room to another. There must a lot of confusion between the newborn sister and the breast she was attached to.

Spring 1992

MR: In a session from next March, Enrico says 'I went out with my friends at the weekend. It was a real positive thing. I read a page in a book but then noticed I couldn't think of what I was reading.

I had impressions, subtle thoughts without realising them; I thought of my friends, I felt fragments of thoughts. Once again I thought of the pain at that time.'

I said they may be fragments to stop the feeling of pain.

He replies: 'Yes, like a real physical thing, I felt something in my stomach, it's something that comes from inside … I've lost my concentration. I feel my head is heavy: my thoughts are heavy and are adrift.'

DM: There's a tendency towards a sort of psychosomatic thing when experiencing passion.

MR: I suggest that when he describes such thoughts and watches their movement and together with me looks at their shape and features, these could become more bearable and comprehensible. He replies: 'Yes, that's right' (but his response is too bland and I wonder if the thought I pronounced isn't too abstract). 'It's never as one thinks. It's like separating yourself from a mirror. It's easier to lie to myself when I'm alone. Today I felt awkward about people I met on the way to the session.' (I think he might have felt transparent and awkward feeling that others were staring at him, but for the time being I add nothing.)

In the first session from the second week of April, Enrico says: 'Last Sunday instead of going out I stayed at home. I did nothing, read some poetry by Baudelaire and a literary essay on Joyce's *Ulysses*. But all this is digging up old history again because I've already read all this. For instance at high school, I learned this page of the essay nearly by rote, actually it was one or two pages, which took me a whole day. I kept going back and forth. Either in bed, or between the bed and the couch, which really makes no difference. I spent the whole day with the book in my hands.'

DM: This is no doubt the story of an adolescent who makes use of the book as an alibi to conceal to himself the fact that he's masturbating. This is the fantasy of masturbating happening.

I suspect he refers to something he didn't say, that is the last chapter in Joyce's novel with Molly's monologue on sexual desire and Joyce's ideas about feminine sexuality; he's reflecting on and trying to understand just this feminine sexuality, although he won't admit it either to himself or to the therapist; he'll never allow himself to admit it.

When Enrico spoke of the monster (in the first dream) again he is certainly confronting the matter of masturbation, with the fear of being caught unawares by his parents. The monster could also relate to a sort of sexual activity with his younger sister, and again to being caught by his parents.

Earlier on Enrico spoke about despair and now a clearer picture is emerging, that is compulsive masturbation; we've moved from ruminating to compulsive masturbation, we've seen this passage take place.

In the course of a normal development the movement would have been from ruminating to fantasies of masturbating, then to dreams related to the analyst and thus to material susceptible of being analysed.

There is a feeling that someone is somewhere – be it Baudelaire, Joyce or someone else – who understands women and their sensitivity and who could teach him something about them.

MR: I ask whether he remembers what the novel is about.

He says, 'I remember the structure of the novel. I didn't study it all but just learned certain sentences and phrases.' He talks about the novel's structure and how the hours relate to episodes linked in some way with Homer's *Odyssey*. 'Each episode relates to a different part of the body: to sound, sight, etc. It's also full of symbols: earth, mother, horse etc. I also remember the novel is structured in different styles and ways of speech. While reading *Epiphany* I tried to identify these elements. I believe I wanted to keep my thoughts busy, stop them from straying away.'

I said, 'It might have been an attempt to stay inside yourself "critically", that is with your brains. Perhaps you tried to keep your thoughts, feelings and parts of your body together, fearing they could break into fragments and head off somewhere on their own.'

He says, 'Yes, as in Baudelaire's poetry; it's always been a sort of Bible to me. I carry it in my pocket all the time. Today too. It's like an amulet but also pure pleasure. Interest and pleasure, and with it I feel less lonely in the afternoon. But then, as with Joyce, it becomes an obsession: I'm left with a feeling as though I'm going to be questioned about it next day, and worry about forgetting the details of what I've read. I had to keep the piece of paper open where I'd taken notes to be coherent. When I went to sleep I had to leave another book open.'

DM: I suspect books could conceal his masturbation fantasies. He had to keep the book page open as he lay to sleep with his mind full of masturbation fantasies.

MR: He continues: 'Today I have this physical sensation my head is swaying. I reread what I'd read, was happy to see that I remembered it well but later felt my head was in pieces as thoughts ran freely and randomly in all directions. My brain is physically swinging, I feel it spinning. Like when I went around in circles this morning out on the street. I was afraid of going back home. When I eventually went back, I started putting the music records in order again.'

DM: The word 'head' which spins freely can easily be replaced with 'penis'. It's as if Enrico were saying: 'I was about to ejaculate and my head was confused and obsessed on the way back home.'

MR: Enrico then talks at length about going to see the Canova exhibition the previous Saturday. I ask him if he thinks anything could explain his feeling unwell the following day. He says, 'I was really attracted by the statues, particularly by *Cupid and Psyche*, their embrace is more than human.'

DM: But he's forgotten the story of Cupid and Psyche is actually a tragedy!

MR: He says he bought a picture of the statue and whenever he looked at it he felt strange (he then describes the statue lovingly). 'Their faces look as though they were alive and talking; the two souls fused into one another. Their love warms one's heart.'

DM: The statue of Cupid and Psyche represents a beautiful fact which however turns into tragedy; something gets denied, which Enrico refers to differently. He identifies himself with the divine Eros, who concedes his love to a quasi-human being and he does it condescendingly. He is then rebuked for such condescension, for being an inadequate lover. This does not correspond with the lover's ideal. This is clearly expressed in Enrico's words when he says of himself: 'Whatever I do does not go down well, there's egoism …'. Certainly all this has to do with his fantasies of masturbation which begin with the idealisation of a love relationship, soon however get denigrated, and perhaps result in an untimely ejaculation. Maria expresses her disapproval, her reprimand, her disappointment in Enrico and everything is thus transformed into a failure.

He is moving towards the problem of how to establish an object relationship, and his capacity for love emerges but is always characterised by egoism and egocentricity. It's almost as though Enrico puts himself in relation not to the woman he loves but to himself and his need to be loved. Enrico is changing his way of relating through the way he regards Joyce, Baudelaire and the analysis. The therapist is the person who can provide him with power and virility, qualities which will make him irresistible in a woman's eyes and which will enable him to relate with someone. First among these with the analyst himself.

Therefore there is a movement from being an isolated boy, enclosed within himself, ruminating about things, to a boy with fantasies of masturbation, who actually masturbates and who has idealised his capacity to love. The existence of object relationships can be seen through this, and in this sense the possibility of change, the possibility of being able to love.

MR: This session was a week later.

Enrico says he has been with a friend who is 'more or less' conscripted. 'He's my best friend. We spent a nice day together, nothing particular. That night, though, I was unusually anxious, slept little and very strangely. I was afraid of being alone. I heard harsh voices of disapproval, they wanted to convince me the day had gone badly. Then the voices became fragments, like uncontrollable fireballs… I had to turn on the radio. It was like hearing a voice from within myself. They are voices which originate from the ideal I've made of myself. It was the voice of the sober, virtuous person I wished I was, the voice of religion, of God, but always voices of mine. The voice scolded me for being selfish and many other things, whatever I've done so far. Now I doubt everything about myself. At times the voice gets louder, becoming unstoppable.'

I fail to understand the appearance of this superego as an external or internal voice which begins to criticise him. Such a state lasted until the beginning of summer. Then his parents decided he should apply for a study grant and leave for Britain 'to learn English.' I thought, they treat him like a parcel: they

send him away without caring about interrupting the therapy, a fortnight before the summer break. At any rate, when
Enrico comes back this phenomenon of voices seems to have
disappeared.

DM: Let's follow the precise order of events …

MR: Enrico tells me: 'I controlled the voices by writing things
down, perhaps a poem, on paper; I wrote them. The images
referred to the morning, initially beautiful but soon turned into
hell with flames devouring the light and then only fragments
of flames remained. Then I walked towards a girl or boy friend
carrying a heart; there was a cathedral, its bells clang horren-
dously, announcing my own death. There was my heart and
woods full of wolves where thieves and merchants took shelter;
love seemed to me the only rescue. No doubt love can help, but
not wholly, entirely, as I believed it would. Putting all this into
words helped me silence the voices.'

DM: This is the best situation: his idealisation is falling apart,
into pieces, and love as an object is taking the place of egocentricity. His attention is now focusing on the object rather than
on himself as the wonderful lover. The analyst is now the object
of maternal transference, a mother not entirely happy with her
son for how he's treating her breast. He is doing it condescendingly; love is offered to him but he expects to be adored. Instead
he gets critical remarks. He's not making the best of the analysis,
he doesn't listen, and doesn't allow himself to be helped. He gets
lost in these idealisations which are however falling apart. The
voices he hears are the analyst's voices, the maternal superego
dissatisfied with his behaviour because he's not co-operating
with the analysis.

MR: I now remember that at first he'd bring me the fee in
an envelope with a short note from his mother, something like
'with much gratitude, doctor'. I used to think the gesture, the
note expressed his wish to talk about his mother (he usually
never talked about his family or his parents). Such an interpretation of mine didn't result in what I'd expected in the following
sessions; that is, the fact he didn't talk about his family had
nothing to do with this and no further handwritten notes came
with the payments.

One time when Enrico was ill, it was his mother who called to tell me he couldn't come. Once again I thought, in the following session, his idea was to send his mother in his place. At the end of May his father rang up: 'How are things going? Do you still need long?' I didn't intend to have any contact with his father so I suggested he should contact the doctor who had initially given my name to him. I also added that the noted doctor was being kept informed of the therapy and thus in a position to answer his questions.

As said, I've always been dubious on this very point. However, as I hadn't asked for an interview with the parents at the start of the session, I thought now it was no longer possible.

When asked about this, Enrico preferred to leave it out altogether.

The last week before the summer holiday

Enrico will be leaving for Britain shortly, sent by his parents, a week ahead of the summer holidays.

First session of the week

Enrico usually comes with a timid, elusive look, and a mild smile, never ostentatious. In one session, however, I worried genuinely as he lay down and started talking without stopping; then he looked round and when he turned his eyes toward me I realised he didn't see me; he looked like a blind boy with his eyes open.

'Well, Doctor' (this is how he usually starts talking once on the couch), 'today I'd like to talk about what we discussed last time: I'm dragging behind a dead part of me which makes me suffer. Saturday went well perhaps because the day before we had a good session. But Saturday afternoon another part of me invaded me, that part that makes me do absolutely nothing. Perhaps it was the bad weather, well I don't remember the weather now ... On Sunday, even though I wanted to go out, I spent the entire day half awake, taken over by the voices. They hurled so many accusations that I couldn't make up my mind. I got up from this mental drowsiness and eventually went out on the terrace. There I was again invaded by voices from the past and rows. It must have been a way of filling my solitude. It was like being nailed down, I could hardly stand on my feet. On Sunday I did manage to do something, I went to Saint Mark's Square. There were people, but the negative part of me increased the feeling of solitude and estrangement.'

DM: To him Saint Mark's Square looks ugly because he sees couples everywhere …

MR: He continued, 'I was afraid the rows, the arguments would follow me back home but then I remembered the record which helps me stop the emptiness. Back at home I listened to it and so I could fall asleep. This morning the voices once again got together to remind me I'm a failure, I cannot be strong and I have no direction. As I came here they ceased a little. At home I kept the radio on, tried doing some physical exercise. I wish I could have gone to the beach, perhaps this would have also made the voices die down. I watched TV but I kept having negative thoughts.'

I ask him to tell me more about the rows.

'They were my former teachers of Latin, maths and chemistry. But the problem was with geometry and how we were asked to study, how he treated my friends, how he taught, how he talked about the subject.'

DM: In point of fact he's arguing with his parents rather than his teachers, he's blaming them.

MR: In fact he hardly speaks about his parents, and when he does only obliquely. His parents, I believe, sometimes go away leaving him alone at home for long periods of time.

DM: Here also his egocentricity appears to dominate all the rest. Excepting a few short breaks filled with solitude, sexual excitement – which makes him masturbate and causes the depression and the voices which persecute him.

But the characteristic that emerges in Enrico is the total lack of interest in what he does, his school subjects, his parents and even the analyst himself. This is a picture one normally encounters in an adolescent between fifteen to sixteen years of age; but he is 22 to 23, already too big to fit such a picture.

Participant: Theoretically speaking, I've always linked self-eroticism with egocentricity, with self-eroticism being the driving perspective and egocentricity the structural one. I gather from what Dr Meltzer is saying that self-eroticism indicates the state of the relationship on a fantasy level and egocentricity as the prevalent one at moments of non-masturbation.

DM: Yes, certainly it's a personality divided between being a young man in the latency period, doing well at school, getting good marks, being a good boy, and a pubertal boy who gets impressed by erotic ideas and fantasies, so he masturbates and attracts the anger of others for his behaviour. Since these two modes cannot co-exist, they contradict one another. The pubertal boy prevents him acting like a latency boy who is obedient and does the work expected of him.

In my view it's the masturbatory part that prevents the good part from winning over, working and going ahead; this masturbatory part is very egocentric, so much so that he can't satisfy his objects. On the other hand these objects of sexual desire are angry with him and show him contempt and disapproval precisely because of his egocentricity, which in a boy at fifteen awakens along with the desire to get flattery and admiration for his penis.

A boy at his age is not interested in a woman as partner in a sexual relationship but as someone who should admire his penis. This attitude goes back to the initial stage in a baby's development, when a baby is adored by his mother and he expects his mother to adore him, especially his little penis. I suspect Enrico's mother truly adored him and his penis only up till the arrival of his younger sister.

At this point the technical question consists in making him see that he isn't putting himself in a right relationship with the analyst. That is, he wants to present himself as a poet, a writer on a par with Joyce, instead of showing the need he has to receive help from the analyst.

This boy's central problem is this: egocentricity! The kind of egocentricity one sees in youngsters at fifteen who believe they are an object of real love. The same thing occurs when girls manifest vanity and boys exhibitionism.

MR: In the session, Enrico continues: 'I associate all this with boredom although geometry was an easy subject and I got good marks. I even remember the page numbers.' (He pauses briefly for the first time in session.) 'As I was lying on the bed I kept thinking about this other me which nails me down, forcing me to watch the passage of time, about my mental attempt to bring in some order, of feeling I'm divided in different parts while trying to hold them united within me, and then the pain and solitude. I meant to tidy my room and take a few things to the cellar but even if one part of me was planning something the other parts were all over the place and it was impossible to move. I felt all the doors inside me were open and voices passed through them.'

I sum up what he's been saying in the session and add that geometry is about organising spaces and parts which come up against one another, which don't come together. He spent a long week end on his own and now is asking me to perform better professionally. He wants me to explain how to put things together. How to get rid of what is not needed and to help him think, reflect.

He says: 'It was the record I was listening to – Bob Dylan. To me it was the calm in the midst of the storm. It was like searching other lost times, the past, the moments of happiness before the onset of difficulties. I was trying to figure out why and when all this began. I recall wonderful holidays spent in the mountains in my second year at high school and so on ...'

I suggest he could be worried about how to order his different parts when he, alone, must try to figure out why he feels the way he does. Moreover, he's scared of going abroad, such a long way from this room.

DM: Although Enrico may seem to be opposing the therapist who reprimands him, his impelling need for analysis becomes clearer. Only when he's in analysis does he manage to find come coherence with himself even for an instant and avoid being enslaved or entrapped in this masturbatory part. Only in analysis can he work and establish a certain relationship, whereas on his own he finds himself helpless before these masturbation fantasies.

He didn't plan the holidays in Britain himself, is there anything he'd like to do?

MR: No, absolutely nothing.

DM: It's a sort of 'fait accompli' that his parents have done for him). I remember an adolescent patient of mine left for South Africa abruptly, interrupted the analysis. I came to know about it only two days before he was to leave and he justified himself as follows: 'Well, it was my parents who decided that for me.' This had very negative consequences on the analysis. He too was 21 and up until that moment his parents also had had no influence on him and it was hard to see why they forced him to leave. There is the same situation now with this young man, and this too is an acting-out which must be analysed to establish the responsibility for this decision. Nevertheless, Enrico's parents had already done something similar when they sent him to live with his grandparents …

MR: It now occurs to me that Enrico was at first sent to me like a parcel which I turned down. The second time, though, he tried to contact me, and asked for an interview.

DM: Enrico might have had fantasies of being swarmed and besieged by hordes of young girls in England who were on the lookout for this young man from Venice.

This interruption will certainly have no catastrophic consequences, such as a psychotic crisis, but it does represent a step backwards, a standstill. And Enrico will keep reprimanding the therapist for getting rid of him, for letting him leave for England. The same happened with my patient, but unlike you I made genuine, serious complaints about it to him and on his return he kept criticising me for not having done enough to stop him leaving.

We mustn't believe all the stories this adolescent tells, as when he says he spends the entire day idling in bed reading Baudelaire or listening to Bob Dylan; no doubt he keeps masturbating. It's as if he wanted to place the therapist in the position of one of his parents who closes one eye, doesn't want to know and simply says: 'Poor thing, he can't do anything about it.' He tries to defend himself against such self-erotic fantasies, and is looking for parental figures to discover his secret and control him. Therefore, it's necessary to eliminate the secrecy shrouding this matter, for otherwise he'll continue being tormented by the voices coming from his demanding, severe superego which keeps criticising, ridiculing and humiliating him. It's necessary to unveil these things for a deeper analysis and to eliminate the voices.

This must be treated naturally, like something that cannot be avoided or put off. If by any chance a pubertal boy says 'no, no, I never do it', it's a way of splitting your attention, as though he didn't know that in fact this was the real thing.

MR: He says: 'In England anything can happen, I'll always be on my own. I don't know if music will help me through it. It's a good experience but I find it difficult to meet new people.'

(At that moment I reflect he won't get psychotic, but he could well get ill, catch a mild illness such as a cold.) 'The positive voices are saying that things can go well. But when leaving, when I'm outside the house, I'll be feeling outside of my life …'

I told him I thought perhaps he needed to be reassured that when he felt 'outside of his life' I'll be keeping this house intact so that he can come back and find I've looked after his things properly (at the same time I imagine I could give him my holiday phone number, but I hesitate).

'The house is a bit of myself and travelling is a way of seeing if the myself-house is strong enough and if it'll resist.'

(I'm relieved not to have yielded to the idea of giving him my phone number.)

DM: Your not disagreeing with his parents' decision allows him to think of you as their accomplice. I'd have worried about him and would have thought it important to let him have my phone number to contact me, but I don't agree that this would all have been useful as a test of strength for him.

Second session of the week

MR: Enrico starts the session saying he had a good day, he accompanied a friend who had to do his final exams at high school and then went cycling with his father. Doing sports and spending time in the open air, he notes, helped him control the voices: 'The worst thing is when I must make small decisions and feel scattered in tiny bits; as I got home yesterday I was shaking with fright they might come back.'

He feared he wouldn't be able to set a barrier against their invasion, something he had succeeded in doing during the session.

'I kept the TV on all night long, the pain nearly gone ...'

I ask him to talk more about his pain.

'When I lie down to sleep all the voices come back and start accusing me.'

Because when alone and when doing sports he wants to masturbate, and then he feels as if spied on and under attack.

'When I do sports I start hearing voices and I lose my sense of calm.'

I say that sports helps him see his body as whole and articulated; he adds, 'and to feel alive ... It's sometimes a desperate attempt. Sometimes I feel I need it, like a sort of medication, to block the voices.'

Participant: Could these be actual hallucinatory voices?

MR: Sometimes he describes them as 'things that come from my inside', but other times they seem to come from outside and do not depend on his will.

DM: I believe his description of the voices is a poetic way of expressing what he feels inside – poetic in the psychoanalytical sense of the word. I don't see anything particularly ill or serious in this young man; rather, I see him in his period of latency and fighting to make his way into puberty. He's very inflexible and tries to avoid adolescence by all means, tries to live beneath it, to pass through it inadvertently and at one point emerges into view as already having a degree, with consolidated achievements, a job, marriage, a solid economic position in the 'doll's house' that I referred to.

Let's look at the dream with the monster: I have described the scene with the cat and the mice in hiding and have linked this to the state of the analysis, to his intention of seeking cover owing to the fear of being found out in his self-erotic practices. I interpret the monster as the incumbent superego which rebukes him for these things.

Participant: I had the impression they were intellectual 'sayings'.

DM: His ruminating is useless, circular, at the service of fantasies of grandiosity and egocentricity.

Participant: Enrico's speech sometimes sounds psychoanalytical – 'one part of me against another part' and so on; could he be reading psychoanalytic books without telling the analyst, or might he have stolen the analyst's language?

DM: Probably it's simply that he hears the analyst talk of one part and another, without relating it to an actual splitting process; he may be making use of these terms also to mix up these responsibilities a little.

Participant: You've said that under similar circumstances you'd have given him your phone number.

DM: Yes, because interrupting the analysis without making a real proper decision on one's own responsibility, but simply from passivity towards his parents who are responsible for this interruption, would have worried me, in terms of a possible panic attack. So I'd have given him my phone number because I'd have wanted him to know, when he felt the need, where to find me and contact me. To tell the truth, patients hardly make use of it.

Participant: Would you have given him the number where you'd spend your holidays or a telephone appointment on a certain day?

DM: I'd have given my home number, there's no reason for keeping it secret. My letterhead has both my home and office numbers. I certainly wouldn't have given him the holiday number, except for an extremely serious case. The analyst shouldn't bear responsibility for his patients during the holidays too. In case of an emergency, a state of severe anxiety or hospitalisation, I'd have given a colleague's number.

When Enrico talked about doing sports, it was obvious he was trying to control his masturbation. It may not be clear, from a certain psychoanalytical perspective, why masturbation control should be the focal point for the patient's attention and preoccupation. Only when we come to the point of understanding the relevance of the process of masturbation to the patient's mental state, will the harm and danger likely to derive from this process become clear. It is the psychic process we are looking at – not just the act in itself, but its meaning.

MR: Enrico continues to talk about his disturbed nights, his divided self, his dead part and his attempts to keep himself whole. [*reads*]

> *Analyst:* The question is how to deal with the dead part and you don't know how to do it. You don't know whether you should leave it inside me or make it come to life with my help. But keeping it is unbearable.
>
> *Enrico:* I feel more united when the two parts come to agree with you and manage to live side by side; then I no longer feel drowsy and am now listening with great attention, for then the thinking part overrides the other. However, I often sense this heaviness and discomfort, especially when I'm alone.

DM: It's interesting to observe the succession of such moments of transference and countertransference, the feelings of drowsiness and alertness. Still, bringing out the term masturbation has finally made him reflect on it.

Participant: What is his unbearable part: the dead part or the excited part?

DM: At this point I can't tell if it's psychoanalytical poetry or some unconscious experience; if it's the dead parts or no 'parts' at all, in the fully psychoanalytical sense of the term: for that means defining the parts. Serious evidence of splitting may also exist but it is not clear enough yet.

Third session of the week

MR: For the past month and a half we have been meeting four times a week. Enrico says he's feeling more at peace and has made a number of decisions: he went to the beach and had a haircut, although shortly afterwards voices returned to remind him of his ugliness and he shut himself in his room 'as though it were a cave'.

> *Enrico:* I've even written about a fictional woman friend met at a place where there were masks, skulls and skeletons.
>
> *Analyst:* It looks like you feel much calmer and trustful with

regards to putting your parts together in my company. Even if in the process skulls, skeletons and whatever else inside you may come out and frighten you. Nevertheless you want to leave these things here, with me, and not take them with you when travelling.

Enrico: Yes, I feel much better also because our sessions are closer together now.

Analyst: You remember the dream of the monster that appeared at a certain time and from which people sought to hide.

Enrico: The monster might be the outside world that I see as hostile, where voices are concentrated … I remember a poet talking about the false world, but that was precisely the world he couldn't attain. I don't mean to compare myself to that poet but I can't say that the entire world is bad. At any rate I have a life that is going ahead but I only have torn ragged pieces, parts of that life. I don't understand what life is in its entirety. Others have a sense of order but I don't. My sister, for instance, is happy with what life offers her: parties, friends. I don't know if that's what I want. For the time being I prefer music.

DM: He's really right in saying this. He certainly can't be an adolescent in the true sense of the word because what he wants is not the world of parties, friends and normal sexuality; he has more grandiose aspirations which he is not yet able to formulate. We don't actually know what the monster represents: whether it is the superego, or a part of the self, or the penis, or the world of adolescents who accuse him of being strange, perhaps a little mad, at any rate distant and a world of his own.

What does emerge more clearly is his perception of being different, of not belonging to the same group and same world as his peers; this is shown by his saying he doesn't wish to join that life, the parties, that is to belong to a world characterised by such participation, friendships, studies, and so on. He says he prefers Baudelaire and Bob Dylan; he isn't yet able to do without his omnipotence.

It may be too soon to tell if this is a boy in latency, obsessive latency, or a boy whose grandiosity and omnipotence stop him from being a normal adolescent, with all the problems linked with adolescence. Or whether this is the case of a psychotic, a sort of borderline personality with grave problems of splitting, living in a claustrophobic world that is clearly distanced from the outside world.

What we can be sure of is that this is a boy who was a good latency child but who cannot tolerate becoming an adolescent like the others. One thing is certain: the problems will not be resolved unless the matter of masturbation is openly discussed.

Participant: Is there any difference, in this case, between real and intellectual masturbation?

DM: These two go hand in hand in the case of intelligent youngsters who might be masturbating physically and intellectually simultaneously. These are often highly gifted boys, maybe almost geniuses, who can actually write poetry, or apply themselves to some other activity, without the need for much study. In Great Britain, I've come across many similar cases; the crisis befalls such young people just when they start college: boys who have had a brilliant high school career become aware when they start university and leave their parents' home for the first time that perhaps they are not brilliant at all.

And the road this boy has chosen: engineering. But apparently he's more inclined to arts and literature. Enrico is sensitive but in only one direction, along a single line: he follows the choices marked by his family and at a certain point he explodes with his excitement or desire which manages to induce a mental opening in him, but this is immediately drowned by his obsessional mode.

Participant: I'd like to know if you agree with four sessions a week.

DM: It all depends on what the patient wants. He said it was ok for him to have short intervals between the sessions, so it's all right. I take the view that in psychoanalysis you need to proceed through experimentation too. So if, for example, the patient asks to change something in the setting you should try to do it. For instance, if he wants to get up later or have more or fewer sessions, any change is potentially welcome. The important thing is to try for some weeks or months, then consider the results and make a decision based on those results; do not decide *a priori* whether changing the setting is good or bad. Meeting one's patients four even five times a week is a nice and efficient way of doing analysis; but two to three sessions a week are enough, the minimal amount; any increase is done for the pleasure of doing it.

MR: My patient hasn't been able to pass other exams and the likelihood of military service is approaching. In the mean time he's expressed an interest in the civil service and in cultural heritage.

DM: Is there any reason for avoiding conscription?

MR: I haven't suggested the civil service to him. I worried that if the analysis was interrupted he might fall to pieces. When he mentioned the civil service I interpreted it as a way to not interrupt the analysis.

[*Dr Meltzer inquires about the military service in Italy.*]

DM: How long have you had him in analysis?

MR: It's been a year now.

Participant: Isn't there a danger his parents might intervene to bring the analysis to an end?

DM: Certainly, his parents are intrusive. Adolescent patients must defend themselves against their parents' interference. For instance, the analyst's decision to not have a direct interview with his father, asking him to see a colleague instead, was sensible and right. Similarly, it has helped to raise the question about his mother's handwritten notes, sent inside the payment envelope. The therapist should have said 'Tell your mother not to send me love messages.'

Participant: If the parents are not told about the rules and not prepared in advance for the length of the analysis, doesn't this increase the likelihood of their interference?

DM: There is nothing that can stop the parents' interference if they don't see positive developments in their son. Or they experience the therapy as a guarantee that their child won't go down dangerous routes such as homosexuality or drug addiction. If this happened, the parents would be the first to reproach the analyst for allowing it.

If it were child analysis, collaboration with parents would be necessary; it's the children themselves who expect that communication between the analyst and their parents to take place. But for patients in puberty or adolescence, the principal factor is respect for intimacy: recognising the fact that analysis is a private matter, and the patients must defend this privacy.

Generally when patients break off an analysis this is due to external reasons (the times, work, their partner's antagonism); such a decision very rarely happens spontaneously as they wish to leave open the possibility of returning to the relationship. One of the likely reasons which have made patients I've had abandon their analysis has been the moment when they felt their own grandiosity and idealisation come under threat; they couldn't tolerate this and preferred to interrupt the process.

In the case of a continuing analysis, there is a point at which certain symptoms and anxieties are recognisably alleviated. At that point one moves into the analysis of depressive anxiety, the 'threshold of the depressive position'; and at this point the analysis may be abandoned. It is when the patient feels a little like a gambler who, since he's won a hand or bet on another round, wants to challenge himself or chance his hand one more time.

CHAPTER EIGHT

Sleeping at his mother's breast: in the style of Oblomov
(1991)

Hugo Màrquez

This is a case about a 42-year-old man, short, bald, rather stout, and almost invariably clad in jeans and an anorak. He speaks very easily and fluently. He says he's had no sexual relationships with a woman, except for a single time when the erection didn't even last properly. As he is too upset and worried he can hardly sleep. His situation worsened a few weeks ago when it occurred to him he might have cancer in his genital organs, the prostate: one morning he woke up with this fear, went through all the necessary medical tests to ensure there was no organic illness; the doctor suggested he should talk about it with a psychologist. His brothers have been helping him to find a solution to his worries; he rang his younger brother living in Rome to join him and the two went to their eldest brother's house. He discussed his problem with his brothers; they talked at length for three whole days, all three highly upset, talked and talked as they walked up and down the room in order to make him admit he'd had no sexual relationships with a woman.

Donald Meltzer: I don't see why he had to talk about this with his brothers!

Hugo Màrquez: I thought his easy and fluent way of talking could be like living the conversation again as though it were still going on with his brothers; this is perhaps what he believes the weekly sessions should be like.

He goes on to say that earlier on, last May, he had a strange incident. As he woke one morning he felt a sharp contraction in his genitals as though they shrank, his testicles were pulled down and his penis drawn in. He could hardly urinate and consulted a doctor who diagnosed prostiitis. Medically speaking, the question thus came to an end, but he kept thinking about it and 20 days ago woke up wholly convinced it must be prostate cancer. A similar situation had occurred 20 years ago; then he was only 22 but already quite isolated, as he still is, and had felt the same as he did in May. He was alone at home studying philosophy, with just one exam to complete his second university degree, and was feeling very lonely. He was studying and, as he teaches English in a secondary school, preparing his school lessons. Twenty years ago that night his father could no longer provide for his studies in Rome and had asked him to come back home; lying in bed at night he had listened to his father's harsh and severe talk with his mother; his father sounded disappointed in him; at that moment he felt his testicles pulled down and his penis shrank.

He goes back to talking about his feelings since May and describes a feeling as if waves from below surge to his head and press on it; while talking with his brothers he discovered his true fear was going mad, that is losing control over his behaviour. Then he talks about sleep deprivation and how he feels at home; initially he felt great comfort at home, felt protected as he studied and read; home was his shelter, the maternal womb; now, ever since May, home has become a trap and he can't figure out why, adding he can't even sleep there.

I point out that perhaps he keeps awake to hear if there are still conversations like the one he overheard twenty years ago.

DM: This is a correct point!

HM: He says he believes history is repeating itself, but fails to see what could have caused such a repetition; he feels basically he has remained stuck to that night in all these 20 years and has been thinking about that night all the time.

Two years ago his father came to stay at the patient's house to have an operation, and now has to come again for a check-up. He says his father was a labourer who wanted his sons to study and become important people; he's never felt he had a true dialogue or shared common points with his father; his father is severe and taciturn. He has always got on much better with his mother; he likes her mother as she is cheerful and energetic and despite her age (70) she often travels. He says he likes women like his mother but that he is like his father, severe and taciturn.

I think to myself, that's not what he looks like to me at all.

He then notes his worries about his sleep deprivation and the period of disinterest in establishing contact with people that he had before May, adding he's fully aware of what's been happening to him.

DM: The first impression the patient makes is that he intimately identifies himself with his brothers; all three brothers are very much linked to one another. It's the first time I've dealt with such a case, for one doesn't speak willingly with one's own brothers and sisters about mental disorders.

I have the impression that these three brothers represent their father's genitals: two of them his testicles and the patient himself the father's penis in such a concrete way that when he grows afraid his penis shrinks and the testicles sag; the brother-testicles who 'come down' to talk when he – the penis – encounters problems. As his brothers represent their father's testicles, they are 'good' testicles. When he makes his confession to his brothers of not having had sex with a woman, these two seem to be saying: 'But we've provided you with so much good sperm and you, what have you done with it?' The patient seems to be answering with 'I've wasted it.' This is precisely what his father is likely to say to him if he came to know it, as when he once said in Rome: 'But I've given you all that money and you, what have you done with it?' Both he and his brothers are regarded as part-objects, as an extension of their dad; now if we question his personal identity, he actually has none of his own but is part of that entity which consists of three brothers who in turn constitute a part of their father's body.

As for that well-known conversation of 20 years ago, it looks as if the patient has taken it as his parents' plot to send him away from home which once was a warm shelter.

Let's consider the child who with his projective fantasies identifies himself with his father's penis; he thus enters into his mother to sleep inside her peacefully. When such children feel that their parents are having a sexual relationship, it's as if a loudspeaker were telling them now they could go into a garage and sleep peacefully; his father's penis places the child inside his mother's body. But when he overhears that conversation, it sounds to him as though his parents are threatening to open the door and throw him out; the void without a name, without an identity, and for the person who has been sleeping inside his mother it leads to madness; to be cast out from the shelter of projective identification into the open space is an unnameable, horrible terror. Bion called it 'nameless dread'.

The patient has no sexual relationships perhaps because he doesn't want his mother and father to have other children and to waste semen. The right word to describe such a state is not 'isolated' but rather 'parasitic'.

Summary of the first year of analysis

At the start of the analysis W. talked about certain symptoms which occur when he comes to the sessions: his head spins, he loses his voice, fears trains, feels his legs become heavy; he's like a complaining, nagging woman. He also talked about encounters with some woman friends, which came to nothing, including a passionate but unreciprocated love at age 25 or 26, to which he reacted with compulsive masturbation.

DM: He's wasting the sperm in revenge.

HM: He says that at present he's not masturbating but after erotic dreams or fantasies often feels a strong urge in bed.

As regards the analysis, at first he accepted it passively with indifference; however, as the noted symptoms disappeared relatively soon, his attitude changed radically to intense devotion. He found he was thinking about his sessions all the time and what he'll be talking about next.

Towards the end of the first month he started suffering from insomnia which still continues. At every session he reports whether he slept or not and there's some implied reproach in his way of speech. We discover that as a little boy when his father came to wake him at night to take him to the bathroom, he'd caress his penis to help him pee.

He feels he's got absolutely nothing to do with the world's violence, and that he's safely sheltered in his superior intellect; his head is still hard as though protected with a helmet, heir to the golden thimble which his aunts would place on his penis and then lift him on top of a table to adore him.

DM: The Dionysian ritual of the cock!

HM: He lives on the top floor and looks down on the world from a distance through a window. He views himself as essentially a good person, not bad like others. His friends confirm this picture of himself, saying he should be less good and generous. He regards all relationships generally as a battle; his father, for instance, used to subjugate his mother but she 'won over' him when he fell ill after a heart attack and ever since, for the past 20 years, has been unable to work.

DM: His fantasy of being, together with his brothers, a part of this representation of their father's genital organs enables him to survive the father figure; it's a manic defence which he needs to give up. He's 'the child inside the breast': comfortable, safe, well and cosy – like Oblomov, Goncharov's character. He has an indestructibility complex, which itself is not indestructible.

Some dreams during the first year of analysis

HM: This is a dream the patient had at the beginning of the second month of analysis. In the first part of the dream, *he's in a hospital holding some files in his hands in front of the nurses' lodge. A man standing before him with his back turned asks the nurse to hand him an encyclopaedia on medicine; this man suffers from throat cancer and tells the nurse he wants to know how one dies. There is also a male nurse who asks this man if he's ever been ill before. The man says no; the nurse tells him it's a pity not to die quickly. Although he can't see his face, the patient knows that this* *man is a colleague and a friend who died from throat cancer two years ago. In the second half of the dream, he is in a city with colonnades where he meets a woman friend, the wife of a colleague. This woman is smiling and very kind as usual but her husband is actually rather a victim, subordinate to his wife; at one point when he turns his back to her, she pushes him from behind and he cries.*

DM: It's interesting to note the contrast between the reaction of crying as in the dream when the woman pushes him outside, and the reaction of compulsive masturbation when a woman turns him down.

HM: The patient had this next dream after coming back from the first analytic holiday. It's a flimsy fragment of a dream as he slept very badly, on and off: *My younger brother and I were in the water in a blue beautiful sea like that in Sardinia; from the top of a cliff someone we could not make out (for we're in a cave) hurls stones into the sea water. There is also a third man, outside the cave in the water, and stones hit him; then my brother and I swim across this cove and come to a tiny but very steep island, like a mountain, and we climb it. The view from above is spectacular: it's sunset, the light is fading, at a distance there's a house in a bay and we think it'd be nice to stay there in peace and quiet. It's getting late, we climb down, and again swim this breadth of water back to the shore.*

DM: This recalls Polyphemus in *The Odyssey* – the giant who persecutes and holds men prisoners in his cave. Until he feels his father's penis is penetrating and ejaculating in his mother, all's well because his mother will sleep soundly, happily, and he likewise in his mother; but if it's him trying to ejaculate and make a woman happy, this is like his pushing his penis inside Polyphemus' cave and he is caught in persecutory anxiety.

It'd be wonderful to go back into the mother-box where all three brothers could live happily ever after. This is what his brothers are apparently suggesting. It's quite a universal fantasy which suggests that before birth we all lived happily in unison in the uterus-box and we all loved one another: the golden sphere of brotherly love which, however, ceases to exist the moment one is born. The patient and his brother play the role of testicles and the third unidentified man represents the brother hit by stones.

HM: These are two dreams he had before the Easter break in 1991:

First dream: *I dreamt I'd left my umbrella in your consulting room. I knocked and knocked but you didn't open; I knocked again, all in vain, but I did see a piece of the umbrella coming from beneath the door; I pulled insistently but it must have got hooked; as I pulled it came out in rags. Still you refused to open the door.*

Second dream: *I dreamt I was in an isolated house in the country with a middle-aged man who was my father; I was a child; the man didn't talk to me but led me inside. He stood by the window and saw something explode in the sky; then he made me understand I had to follow him downstairs. We walked down the stairs through a maze of stones till we came to a shelter with food. Then we went out into the open, I walked beside him; we stopped at a bar where he met other people, I always at his side. We had to bathe in the sea, but first had to negotiate a slope. As we went down I felt the stones and pebbles were loose under my feet and could easily slide, I had to be very careful where to set my feet but managed to get down unscathed. Then I bathed; the water was very warm as if there was a volcano underneath, and my father warned me – I saw columns of smoke rise.*

DM: The volcano is his father's penis. He's wasting his father's sperm.

HM: This is a dream he had before the summer holidays in 1991: *My brothers and I were in a filthy hotel. Then I was inside a white church with very tall arches.*

DM: Rectum and vagina, or inside the breast.

HM: [*continues to relate the dream*]: *I looked up, looking for someone; my younger brother was nowhere to be seen; police officers pointed at the asphalt road with blood stains and remains of a brain; it might have been an accident, but they looked very suspicious, ambiguous.*

DM: In the last dream violence arises against the younger brother who, by not complying with his brothers' rules that they function as a harmonious unity, has a life of his own and therefore does not deserve to be loved; their fraternal love holds only if he accepts being part of this unique entity, otherwise he deserves to be killed violently.

The drama of the younger brother's birth and the patient's immense jealousy are brought into the transference and the patient will soon discover his analyst has other patients.

The three brothers make up a triumvirate who conspire to seek and maintain power; it rests on a very unstable balance and none of the three brothers can implement their power alone. Often two brothers come together to oust the third; it can even come to killing one another just for the sake of this power struggle. There's some visible improvement towards demolishing this triumvirate; its indestructible mask of goodness and generosity is about to crumble. This is evinced precisely through the emergence of violence due to the recognition of the existence of other children, which unleashes intense feelings of jealousy.

My prognosis is that this is not an extremely serious case; this is a form of family neurosis brought about in a certain family culture that is already beginning to disintegrate, and he started analysis before his father's death. In terms of parasitism it is a benign case; he harms no one; the real concern is wasting so many years of his own life. If he were a woman entering analysis at 42, it would have been more serious as this would be towards the end of her fertile period. This patient's only depressive problem is the waste of time. However, he hasn't been a useless, destructive parasite, for he works, has a group of friends who say he is a good man, and so on.

Second supervision – December 1991

This supervision took place two months after the previous one.

HM: I have now realised that W. is regarded as 'the investment of the family' and that they hold him in high esteem, seek his advice, and listen to his views. The patient's identity, as Dr Meltzer noted before, consists in being a part of this family, particularly through his unity with his brothers as a part of their father's body that will live beyond his death – a manic defence mechanism.

DM: This is a very interesting family constellation in which the father seems to have relegated himself to being the baby of the family of twenty years ago.

Recent evolution of the analysis

HM: Since the patient's first holidays back in August, and in particular since we changed the session times at his request (something I did not do immediately but after a few days), he has realised he is not my one and only patient.

DM: How long was the summer holiday?

HM: Four weeks.

HM: As a result, since resuming the sessions, he's been treating me with cold formality and complaining the analysis hasn't alleviated his troublesome sleeping disorder and that he can no longer remember his dreams. He tells me what happened after each weekend at great length, talking about every event as though it were the same, even when talking about his father's chemotherapy.

He seems to be treating me like a stranger: politely but formally. I need to get over this distance or dive into deep interventions unless I wish to stay 'outside'; but he's not too rigid and the emotional tone of the sessions increases in warmth soon after my interpretations. Topics concerning cold, warmth, the sun, freezing fog and so on, and concerning outside and inside – inside the train that brings him to the sessions, scenes out of the train window, inside the house, outside through the window – have now moved to the foreground.

W. has changed his job: at a suggestion from a woman friend he has known since childhood he is now a member of a group of four teachers giving tuition to immigrants coming from outside the European Union. He's become the soul of the group and prints the hand-outs to teach 'these blacks', as he calls them affectionately; they need to learn everything from a scratch as the pupils are mostly mother-tongue Arabic and don't know how to read and write the Latin characters.

DM: They are being taught Italian or English?

HM: Italian.

In this regard, the group are given a completely free hand by authorities to manage the formal organisation and the course content; W. is enthused by his choice of contemporary issues such as social criticism, environment, life in big cities, which allows him to step out of the monotony of official teaching curricula.

DM: Back to 1968.

Participant: Four as in his family.

DM: Minus the father.

HM: He calls this group of teachers to which he belongs 'the gang of four'.

Participant: Like the historic one in China.

DM: He'd have been around 20 at that time.

HM: He's absorbed in his job and his pupils gradually turn into big mouths that need constantly to be fed in order to stay shut. He feels he thus 'avoids depression and stays on an even keel'. The family has also started to talk about the expected death of his father; W. can no longer stay in his father's house as they 'may want to talk'; therefore he spends his days mostly outside and thinks about what to do at his new job.

DM: Do we know whether his father had a heart attack before or after 1968?

HM: He explained his father had it after 'the famous conversation' between his parents when he came back from Rome. The patient was made to return to the family house after a year at the Physics Faculty in Rome, without sitting an exam, and his father told his wife 'W. is good for nothing'; he was made to give up studying physics and the following year he started studying for a language degree in a nearer town. He stopped his physics studies in June and his father had a heart attack in December.

DM: So he's been in analysis now for a year and a quarter. When did this group of four come together?

HM: Last October.

DM: Because we didn't hear about them last time. They are newly set up.

A recent session

HM: The three weekly sessions are on Wednesday, Thursday and Friday. Before W. took up his new job, we'd meet on Tuesday, Thursday and Friday; but as he wanted to change the hours I also had to move the sessions to another day. At first the patient seemed to accept this but now he has been complaining as the intervening weekend is too long for him; perhaps I could resume the initial order of sessions from January next year.

His sleeping disorder continues. He doesn't feel depressed yet doesn't know how to describe his mood which is anything but positive. The daily routine and ongoing inertia disturb him. He tries to persuade himself he is much better than he was a year ago and that this is quite significant. He talks about Christmas gifts in a similar manner: he'll buy a brooch for his mother as he does every year. [*reads:*]

> **Analyst**: You're pinned to your mother's breast.
>
> **Patient**: I thought I was far away, distant, not stuck onto her!
>
> **Analyst**: I don't consider you a mummy's boy but rather, as being all one with your mother, which prevents you from feeling things and confirms your impression that everything is monotonous, flat. Just as when you start talking about everyday events in great detail, it's as if you were trying to make us all one and the same.
>
> **Patient**: I'd like to be transparent, I want my mind to become transparent.

DM: It's true, it *is* transparent. You can see him inside his mother's breast! You'll probably find his mother is very worldly, knows everything that is going on around her, the neighbours' business and so on. She is not only lively but talkative, exchanging news and gossip with all the neighbours. This is a caricature of his mother's way of presenting the world to him – news of the outside world which he then recounts in the sessions.

HM: I said to him, by doing this with your internal space, your personal lived experience will disappear too.

Participant: It has struck me that the patient didn't want to stay in his parents' house as he feared his father might say things against him, and then I wondered if he might not have the same fear during the sessions, for you might tell him things that would hurt him.

DM: What he's afraid his father will talk about is a repetition of his father's anger at him, blaming him for pushing him out of the mother's bed as it were. In a certain sense he hears Hugo's interpretations as complaints. So the technical problem is really to find the maternal transference: the patient is quite insistently keeping him in the position of the father who has been pushed out of the intimacy between the brothers and the mother.

One of the things I think would correspond to the maternal transference is the arrangement about the fees he pays you, which probably will turn out to have a similar significance to the brooch which he yearly gives his mother. Also the way in which he reports things to you, though as you say it has the quality of being like a news bulletin with very little feeling in it, it's probably true that, as he says, he wishes his life to be transparent to you. And this is part of the maternal transference. He's the good boy who comes home from school and tells his mother everything that went on there – in this boring, mechanical way.

It is one of the difficulties of the male psychoanalyst; the paternal transference is always very obtrusive, because of the fact of his masculinity. It is necessary to find all the little evidences of the maternal transference, in order to bring this image of the maternal object forward in the analysis. It takes a lot of work usually.

Second recent session

HM: During the first half hour of this session he managed to fall asleep.

DM: It is generally true of the person who suffers from insomnia; it's like the fat person who says she never eats anything. It is impossible for people to survive with less that three or four hours' sleep a day. But it does represent a psychic reality: they are deprived of sleep because like a child they are constantly monitoring the sounds from the parents. That is what they are suffering from. Part of the insistence that they haven't slept is the insistence that nothing has happened in the parents' bedroom.

This sort of thing goes back to early infancy where the anxiety of the child, the moment the mother is not in sight, is immediately transferred to the ear – to listening and mapping her activities, what she's doing in the kitchen, in the toilet, the bedroom.

A constant monitoring of the mother to keep contact with her. It goes back to the first six to eight months of life. It continues later in childhood: if the mother goes out of the house the child is constantly thinking of her: now she's walking down the street, now she's in the butcher's shop... etc. Then of course this monitoring contains a prediction that 'now I will begin to hear her footsteps', and as soon as they appear, it has the significance of having control over the mother.

The listening out, and the listening in, have two different significances. In so far as this man is an inhabitant of the breast, he is in a position to listen and to look in both directions. These get divided into nocturnal and diurnal listening: at night he is listening in, during the day he is looking and listening out. At night he is listening anxiously and controlling omnipotently by his knowledge of what is going on: listening to the different compartments within the mother: the sexual compartment, the genital compartment, the rectal compartment. Listening for evidence of sexuality, and listening for crimes (in the rectum). During the day, the listening and looking out is from this position of Oblomovian detachment: looking with cynicism and pessimism at the stupidity and brutality of the outside world.

Now the spirit of 1968 which holds sway over the 'gang of four' is a mixture of communism and Christianity: that the first shall be last and the last shall be first. That is, the poor black children in the rectum shall be made white. The immigrants – Italian style!

HM: While he was sleeping in the session he had the following dream: *I was driving up a rocky headland. It was a wide smooth road; I drove up along the edge and could look below at the rough sea. I stopped and people in bathing suits just dived into the sea nonchalantly and talked about their own diving experience; I thought it was so dangerous! A light wind, a breeze pushed me to the edge of the ravine, I had to crouch and creep as I held on to the soil with my nails. I managed to get into the car and kept driving up the road. I got to a clearing where few Americans were having a picnic on the ground. I got into the car and started driving up again but I didn't know where I was going, for I found myself in my bed in my grandfather's house, and my brother came to wake me, telling me*

three immigrants had been killed and that he, the head of the immi-
grants, was joining a demonstration. I stayed in bed. I went out of
the house and all my cousins in their bathing suits were on their way
to the beach and suggested I should also go along but I didn't want
to, so I walked back to the house and lay down to sleep again.

DM: There are different scenes aren't there: first the bathing
scene and his recovering the car; then there's the scene of the
picnicking Americans; then the scene in his grandfather's bed;
then, fourthly, the account of the murders; and fifth, the invitation to go bathing. Five different scenes in this complicated
dream. Does he have a car?

HM: Yes.

DM: OK. Does he swim? Is he afraid of water?

HM: He doesn't like water and almost all his dreams have to
do with water, the sea and the like.

The dream might have started with his cousin's invitation to
join them, or perhaps the whole dream is his thinking about
dangers and the pointlessness of inviting them. I said to him
that I thought the light breeze represented my breath, my drift,
my interpretations; it seems he felt them as a dangerous invitation to do something risky which for others would be absolutely
natural; my interpretations would make him jump so he resists
with terror.

DM [*making a reference to the patient's name, W.*]: In a Walt
Disney film there are two American names, Walker and Wheeler,
which are used in an interesting way to show how a man's character changed when he got into his car, from a peaceful to an
aggressive one. In this dream there is a recurring theme: getting
into and out of a car.

The first scene is about the danger of going out and finding
himself in water; it represents his fear of water. I'd relate the scene
with Americans having a picnic with envy; these are rich people
doing well, whose family life is idealised as they are in televi-
sion; he wishes to be like them. The third scene, I think, relates
to the patient's father and with confronting his father's dying
condition. The fourth scene takes up the anxiety with respect to
what happens inside his mother if he and the gang of four are
not there to help her. And the fifth scene proclaims his decision

never to get out of the mother but to resist any invitation to go out, particularly to resist all sexual temptations.

I think you are right about the light breeze of your interpretations, because this seems to have a terrifying effect on him. But it also means that so long as he's inside the car the wind can blow as much as it likes, it doesn't touch him. It's only when he comes out that your interpretations affect him.

I think that when a patient living in projective identification brings you a dream, this is your best opportunity to catch him and bring him out of it; in this case an interpretation is bound to have touched him.

HM [*resumes account of session*]:

Analyst: Now let's move on with the headland-dream and get to the Americans' picnic, and here apparently your mother's breasts are represented: this is where you eat; they are also high up; that they are Americans has to do with your own first name. Thus, going back to the brooch as your Christmas gift to your mother: obviously she wears it close to her heart, on her breast; you are fastened to your mother's breast and no-one can make you change from that position. But the younger brother who comes from outside the family, an extra-European migrant, evicts you saying: get off, off your mother, now I've come to feast here, which is why you can hate him as much as you hate my interpretations as represented by the three assassinated, non-European migrants (the patient has three sessions weekly).

Patient: My maternal grandmother chose my name; I was her, my aunts' and my mother's favourite; everybody held my grandmother in great respect ...

Analyst: So the headland is 'Olympus'.

Patient: Yes. I remember once when I was three or four, I wanted to buy ice-cream; I asked my grandmother to give me two 5 lire coins but she gave me one 10 lire coin. That's not what I'd wanted.

Analyst: The two 5 lire coins must be your two hands with five fingers with which you might have wished to touch your adored grandmother's breasts and eat the ice-cream there instead of in the ice-cream shop. I also think that the boy on Olympus was pushed off and brought down to earth with the birth of your younger brother, the new favourite, and you ended up with your grandfather and his two drawer-testicles, but you refused to be pushed into being a little boy who has to get into his swim trunks and go to the beach like the rest of his cousins.

DM: That's very imaginative! I'd take the coins more literally because at that age he wasn't likely to know the meaning of five, so wouldn't have had a reference to the fingers of his hand. But the idea of giving two little coins and getting one big one was meaningful to him; and he didn't really believe his grandmother, that the one coin was the same. And from there, you could move to the two nipples versus the one penis for sucking: as if the grandmother was offering him the grandfather's penis which links up with him finding himself in his grandfather's bed. Because there is certainly a homosexual anxiety in this man, related to his femininity and to his feminine identification. But it's very difficult to get at until you can get into the maternal transference and can interpret to him his identification with you as a maternal figure, and his beginning to carry on an analytic practice as it were with his friends.

Was it correct that in the dream it was all male cousins who invited him to the beach?

HM: The atmosphere in which he talked about the dream was as if it had to do with boys' games and tricks.

DM: All boys together.

HM [*resuming*]:

Patient: Even now I don't want to go to the sea with them, so I sleep until late; then I go out for a walk and come back to sleep. Today I was in a good mood.

Analyst: Because in the dream you are not evicted by the interpretations I made yesterday; you cling onto your mum's bosom tooth and nail. However, one can see you're very angry and you'd rather kill than relinquish your position on Olympus.

DM: I don't think the last part is quite correct really. So long as the patient is inside his mother and feels he can organise and monitor whatever happens in there, his anxiety about his mother's survival is greatly diminished. It's only his father outside who is the object of this death anxiety. As soon as he's outside and the group of four isn't inside protecting and elevating these black children, the anxiety about his mother emerges; but that would bring an entirely different type of hypochondria with it.

What introduced this present illness was a prostatitis connected with masturbation and his identification with his father's penis, and the three brothers enacting the fantasy of being their father's genital organs. But his two brothers have gained prominence: they have their own children whereas he hasn't, which is why he feels he is the shrinking penis that gets ever smaller. The configuration of the three brothers wherein he attempts to aggrandise himself by heading north, taking up philosophy studies, becoming a schoolteacher and the one whom everyone in the family turns to and listens to, is a compensation which is gradually diminishing and is being reshaped. It was a compensation for his lack of sexuality but now is being re-established through the 'group of four', which assigns him an important role as a revolutionary, a former 1968 activist. But in fact, the group of four is showing its first cracks: the students are increasingly demanding, yet passive – as in the description of having open mouths – which makes the initiative lose its lustre, its revolutionary significance.

HM: Indeed, this is what's happening to the group. His childhood friend who had initially suggested he should join the project has already grown weary and is now thinking of taking up a training course in Switzerland to work in Africa, and W. thinks he should follow suit.

DM: Now let's consider the balance of the forces operating on him at this point in his life. The dream shows him making little forays outside his position inside the breast, and the anxiety he meets when he goes out, and how he then retreats. The analysis has richly contributed to this new instability.

In a certain sense the dream also represents what happens in the course of a session: he retreats inside, comes out, meets with anxiety, retreats, and so on. Each of these anxieties is worth examining and drawing his attention to: his fear of water, his envy of rich people, his anxiety about homosexuality, his fear of violence, and his inability to be one of the group of masculine people. It all centres really on his masturbation – throwing his seed on the ground as it were.

A dream like this almost lays out a programme of the analytical problems that need to be investigated and resolved before his masculinity can emerge. To be one of the boys means to be equal with his brothers: not to be the penis while they are the testicles, and so on. With a patient like this you are in a race against time. It is essential that these analytical accomplishments be made before his mother dies. Because at the time of his mother's death the only thing that could keep him from becoming manifestly psychotic would be some other woman being like a mother to him, looking after him without expecting sexual intercourse. This is basically what happens to Oblomov.

The central part of the session where he very co-operatively remembers this incident of wanting an ice-cream cone points to something very important: his anxiety that if you don't find nipples to suck from, you have to suck from penises. His anxiety about homosexuality has to be touched on: but this is difficult until the maternal transference is well established in the analysis.

With reference to the light breeze that almost blows him off the promontory: you have taken it in a way that probably carries with it the implication of the paternal transference – of father saying he's too big to be at the breast, he needs to be weaned. Yet you can just as well see it from the perspective of the mother who is irritated by this child who refuses to be fed from a spoon and will accept nothing but the nipples. This is represented by his insistence on asking for two 5-lire coins. I think you have to watch the material attentively for every opportunity to interpret the maternal transference.

Third recent session

HM: Last night he couldn't sleep a wink. He says the previous day his mother told him his blanket was nowhere to be found; the cleaner might account for the loss. He says the previous day one of the immigrants had drunk too much; he lives in a flat without heating. [*reads:*]

Analyst: If the analysis goes on like this I'll be evicted from my refuge and will have to sleep rough so I should get a supply of blankets and find some sort of heating. Perhaps he keeps awake to make sure no brother immigrant comes along.

Patient: Yes, one's coming tomorrow. It's true, I listen to catch the slightest noise: from the flat below, the bathroom on the other side of the wall, trains in the station, refuse collection trucks, cleaning ladies in the block opposite.

Analyst: You seem to have mapped out the outside world through sounds; this is the opposite of what doctors do by placing a stethoscope on a patient's back.

DM: Like radio astronomy. I'm surprised we don't hear anything about smell. Does the patient have a distinctive smell?

HM: He has a sharp smell, almost a stink.

DM: Doesn't he wash?

HM: I think when he's overanxious he sweats a lot and stinks.

DM: This question is explored and written about too little in psychoanalytic literature – the smell that emanates from people depending on their mood; however thoroughly they may clean themselves, whatever they may chew, they keep stinking, and this torments them. This is a significant detail that needs to be noted when presenting the patient. It afflicts them terribly. Partly because they cannot really smell it themselves; it is the same with people with bad breath. They are exquisitely sensitive to how far people stand from them. So he smells bad – that's interesting. You should mention that in your summary.

HM: [*resumes*]:

Patient: That's true. There were some blacks on the waterbus today and I tried to listen to their conversation.

Analyst: Blacks can relate to darkness, to conversations held in the dark.

Patient: Always! Just as I listened to the conversation of my parents from my bedroom 20 years ago. My father was telling my mother I was no good for anything, and I felt my genitals shrink.

DM: These are opportunities for interpreting the transference about what you and your wife, your partner, talk about him; and his worry that you are getting discouraged, that he won't ever accomplish anything in analysis.

This material relates to the anxiety of six-month babies and the way they monitor their mother's movements. They try to sharpen their hearing to capture all the sounds that may come from their mother; the sense of such control from a distance of the mother's movements is to stay in contact with her. This goes on in years, and thus when the mother goes out, the child knows she's now going down the stairs, crossing the street; such monitoring also includes the sense of predicting; 'now she's going up the stairs, coming back, and I'll see her walk in', and this gives the impression of having complete control over the mother. Listening to outside voices or sounds has a significance different from listening to sounds coming from within; in this patient's case who breathes out from inside his mother's breast, the listening is two-fold; it is directed towards outside and inside and divided into daytime and night-time listening; at daytime he watches and listens outwards, at night he watches and listens inwards; at night-time he listens anxiously to and controls with omnipotence what's going on in every compartment of his mother: in her sexual compartment and her rectus compartment. This mode of listening is on the lookout for any evidence of sexual activity and criminal deeds (in the rectus); whereas the daytime watching and listening occur in a fashion similar to Oblomov's, towards trifles and silly things, and the brutality of the outside world, all done at a distance with cynicism and pessimism.

HM: This is an opportunity to interpret to him his fantasies about my conversation with my wife about himself, and to tell him that he may be worried that I get disheartened and disillusioned by him.

DM: The Americans having a picnic must refer to himself watching his brother at his mother's breast. Do you know the names of his brothers? [*No*]. You may be surprised when you find out.

HM: [*resumes*]:

Analyst: Did your testicles become as small as when you were a child?

Patient: Yes, they did.

Analyst: Going back to the dream we talked about yesterday: when you were sent away from your grandmother's and your aunts' Olympus apparently you were thrown down at the foot of your grandfather's chest of drawers, that is you fell between his testicles, which is where you put yourself together again to become the little 'man of the house', your father's and grandfather's penis. Perhaps from then on you felt you had a mandate to represent the family, but from that conversation onwards it looked as though they intended to withdraw the mandate and throw you out again, without a role, like a defenceless child.

DM: At this point you could have mentioned the next baby. He is very co-operative in the sessions.

HM: [*resumes*]:

Patient: Well, that's true. We, all three brothers, were encouraged by our father, who boasted about us as good sons; perhaps it was because we were a humble family. But at the time I was the only one who went to university; my big brother already had a job and the little one was still at school.

Analyst: Picking English studies after dropping out of physics could also be a forced attempt to realign yourself with the world of your grandmother who had given you an English-sounding name.

DM: That's very good. Holding it together. But to go back to the very beginning of the session: he did experience his mother as accusing him of masturbating, getting semen all over the cover. He is really feeling a pressure to get out in the cold. It is more and more clear that he is experiencing you as a combined object: as mother and father talking about him and deciding this baby has to be weaned; so long as you feed him at the breast he thinks he's living inside the breast; and anyhow we want a new baby. You get a picture of a baby who won't accept anything but the nipple and won't have anything to do with toilet training;

he's still wetting and soiling himself – this content baby who refuses to develop.

I think the gap between sessions is too long for him.

Fourth recent session

The patient relates two dreams he had after the last session:

First dream: *I'm wandering in the country at night; I come to a small, unpretentious house, all the windows are lit and people are talking inside; I ring the bell but no one comes to open it and I feel the void within me, no one cares about me; I keep ringing and a friend's wife comes to open it but leaves me standing alone at the door, as though to say 'get on with your own business'. I go in, there are five or six people sitting on the floor and my philosopher friend is reading aloud to them. All the people are friends or acquaintances from his home town and they're writing down names on a piece of paper, as many as they can recall for each letter of the alphabet; they are busy and don't even greet me. All at once they all begin to add the letter W before the names they've already put down on paper – many Ws.*

Second dream: *Again I'm walking in the country at night with a hammer in my hand. After a while I sense there's another man walking behind me, and soon he starts following me. I begin to run and so does he; he too is carrying a hammer; I clamber up an embankment and someone from above tells me to run faster; the man from behind throws an axe at me which strikes the ground behind me. Running on I get to a castle and enter a splendid draw-ing room as big as a museum, all lit up; the people are all well-dressed and I notice a man wearing a bow-tie. I'm still holding the hammer; I look around to see how to get out. There is a large window with small leaded glass panes; I break it with the hammer; the bars behind easily give way to my blows and I go outside as if crossing into another country, as though the window were a frontier and by crossing to the other side I'm rescued.*

DM: That's an extraordinary dream. It's a real claustropho-bic dream; yet in the previous dream he was agoraphobic. The significant thing is that the splendid room is described as a 'museum' – lifeless.

HM: I've noted that in these two dreams he first wandered around outside as if with some vaguely delinquent intention, which was followed by going in and breaking the windows to get out; but I don't see how he got in.

DM: It's the baby's teeth – the axe – for getting in, but then the same implement is used for getting out of the mother's body.

Participant: Here the question of being inside or outside the mother's body is being repeated.

DM: Yes, but for the first time we've seen claustrophobic anxiety. Previously being inside was very comfortable, and aloof, and all the dangers were outside. The significant thing is the museum. Often it is represented as a natural history museum, with all these lifeless models of animals in glass cases.

HM: I didn't notice anything then and so didn't ask him anything or if he made any associations.

DM: It's all right, just the naming of the museum is what's important.

HM: Last Saturday his younger brother, together with his own son, came to fetch his parents to take them to their home; the following day, Sunday, he felt very lonely and very hollow; then he remembered the dream and understood that he'd imagined everyone together like the people in the modest country house in the dream and that his feeling of emptiness was identical to what he'd felt in the dream.

DM: Of course the person following him in his dream is his younger brother.

HM: Then he says he suddenly felt very angry with his mother as she no longer wished to have the old chest of drawers and wardrobe she'd insisted he take to his house, and now when he brought them back she didn't like them at all; the discussion with his mother was very heated and he himself was surprised by the intensity of his feeling. [*reads*:]

> **Analyst**: What I find significant in the second dream is that you are walking in the country at night with a hammer; you're trying to say the dangerous and violent person other man is, the man following you, but it's you who's wandering around at night!

Patient: Yes, that's true. The hammer reminds me of my father's carpenter's workshop.

Analyst: Apparently as you were assembling the old chest of drawers and the wardrobe with a hammer you had this sudden surge of anger against your mother and the rest of your family which you imagined all gathered together without you, as you stood out in the cold. I also think the window in the dream is similar to the entrance of the building where my study is located.

Patient: That's right, it's very similar.

(He insists on the sense of relief he had as he crossed the border into another country where the man behind could no longer follow him.)

Analyst: But if we agree to regard the violence as your own and not that of the other man, then it's you who breaks the law by escaping into another country!

Patient: Well, yes, because in the dream it was like I had got away with it.

Analyst: If the hypothesis is true that the window refers to the entrance of the building with my study, perhaps the dream tells something also about how to avoid being influenced by my interpretations, how to abandon the sessions.

DM: There is nothing unusual about the door in this Venetian setting; it is not likely to be convincing to him to interpret it as a matter of breaking out of the analysis. You would have to come to it after analysing why this museum experience was so claustrophobic that he had to break out of it with a hammer. If you relate this hammer or later the axe to the baby's teeth, then if the baby wants to be weaned, the best way to ensure it is by biting the nipple. This breaking the window or door with the hammer constitutes biting the nipple and forcing the mother to wean him, as if it's the mother's fault that he is kept in such an imprisoned state, being such a baby that he never develops his masculinity. His accusation against the mother comes out in the accusation of having this cupboard brought into the house when she didn't even like it. I would think this window he breaks out of represents the nipple: biting it and breaking out of this relationship to the mother.

I don't think he accuses you any longer of keeping him in the analysis as a claustrophobic prisoner. You are mostly experienced as a combined object – the two parents talking together about how to wean this baby. You can see from the dreams how things have been in a delicate balance: he makes little forays outside, gets frightened, runs back inside. Now suddenly the valency has changed: the inside becomes the bad place, and the outside becomes the place of liberty. That is a turning point really.

Participant: Do the claustrophobic experience and the violence in relation to his mother mean that a separation would be like falling into an endless pit?

DM: This doesn't seem to be a major anxiety; we really haven't met the major anxiety, just a list of anxieties in the first dream, none of which were overpowering, just unpleasant and a bit frightening. Nothing you could call a catastrophic anxiety in defence of which he remains inside. One could only say 'what a comfort-loving baby'; and generally, as of Oblomov, where is his capacity for aggression? And how is it possible to establish masculinity without a capacity for aggression? The capacity to penetrate undoubtedly has its origins in the nails and teeth as penetrating instruments, potential weapons.

It is interesting to see in male patients who become vegetarians a background of a real difficulty in chewing. With all sorts of political and sociological rationalisations, the fact remains that there is a difficulty in aggression and in penetration that shows up just as much in sexual life as in relation to food.

What begins to arise in the transference at this turning point where he has abandoned being inside as a lifeless place, is that he is bound to become aware of your other patients and of a sense of being the failure, the one who has failed at physics and turns to English as an easy second choice. There emerges an acute sense of being 42 and therefore 20 years behind in his social and sexual development. The problem of the masturbation as a waste of his masculinity and his semen is bound to come to the fore of the material.

Fifth recent session

HM: Last night he had a fragment of a dream: *He was driving his old red Renault 5 car up a winding road; it was again night time. He was driving fast and had taken a wide bend, almost running over a woman, the wife of a friend from his hometown; she and this friend were walking along the road but he nearly ran her over. As he kept speeding he heard them say behind 'Look at this one! He sure is reckless! Look how he's driving! We should call the police.' He looked through the rear-view mirror and said 'heavens, they haven't recognised me!' He kept driving fast up the winding road and saw a police car come in the other direction; he feared it might be coming to get him but it didn't stop; then a second police car appeared and this one too passed by as he gave a sigh of relief for having got away with it.*

He says the dream has little worth and talks on in a formal and shallow tone as if talking about everyday matters. [*Reads*:]

> **Analyst**: I believe you're putting it like that so that we should not stop and analyse the dream.
> **Patient**: That's right. I think this too is getting away with it another time.
> **Analyst**: Indeed. The question of the rear-view mirror may refer to me, whether I've noticed anything dangerous or violent in you.

DM: He's once again inside something, but this time not in a place of safety, rather of aggression, a car. As the hammer represented the teeth before, now he has become an aggressive daddy-penis. This dream has the significance of flashing, of publicly exhibiting his erection. And you are the combined object: his mother and father.

HM [*resumes*]:

> **Analyst**: The landscape you describe has also changed: the peaceful sublime Olympian headland is now the winding road going uphill presenting danger and violence.
> **Patient**: That's right. My childhood friend [the sister of the woman who once turned him down; she's also the person who suggested he should join the project with immigrants] is

leaving for Geneva next year to do a training course before going to Africa or some other third world country as a volunteer worker; I think I should also leave as I've come to an end of working as a teacher of children; and the experience I've had with the immigrants seems to be finished too; so I think I'll also leave in order to do something else.

Analyst: This sounds like a threat to interrupt the analysis if I don't stop making interpretations.

Patient: Yes, I thought 'if it works, I'll break it off'; but I also thought of the contrary, if it works why not go on and try to understand things better? But this Africa project is no big deal …

Analyst: I don't think so at all. It's blackmailing me because now you think you're no longer the one who risks being thrown out, left in the cold, which was why you kept track of every single sound at night. Now at night you imagine violent ramblings, and criminal thoughts; your insomnia has completely changed its significance.

DM: You are a bit puzzled as to why this material comes up after you have interpreted the transformation of the peacefulness of Olympus to this tortuous violent masturbation: that contains fantasies of exhibiting his erection in front of all these couples, so the women would all leave their husbands for him – the usual exhibitionist fantasy – even if he ejaculates prematurely and will despise these women.

The patient says this car, the Renault 5, is strong and useful, even though others think it is out of fashion: it is the rationale of the person who picks through the rubbish to find the things that other stupid people throw away – we call it scavenging. The redness of the car probably stands for the erection. Originally it was violence in the mouth; and the baby's teeth (represented by the hammer or the axe) has now changed through projective identification with the father's penis into the aggressive psychology of the exhibitionist.

It is connected with the accusation against his mother that is represented by his bringing this furniture into the house even though she didn't like it. Whereas there is plenty of evidence that the mother eventually did wean him and did have another baby;

and there's the conversation of 20 years ago which showed that both parents were disappointed in him, with his failing at physics.

He accuses you as the analyst-mother of giving him only the leftover sessions, keeping the best times for the others, and of not working hard for him. Whereas in fact you've been working like a dog for him! Such a dream is also worrisome because it is a plan for acting out. It is important to get at it quickly before his starts acting it out.

HM: In the following session he just did.

Participant: As you told the story about his mother insisting he take the chest of drawers and the wardrobe, I recalled the game children play putting pieces of furniture together to make a whole, and then thought he might have blamed his mother because she had forced onto him a combined object.

DM: I think he accuses his mother of imposing a feminine identification onto him. Perhaps she asked him to help her with the new baby, as she didn't have a daughter.

HM: His fantasy is, as he's not married, he's supposed to look after his mother when she becomes a widow – the custom in southern Italy – and he would have to play the bachelor-son.

DM: He is a fairly effeminate man; there is plenty of scope for his motherliness, which probably has been reinforced by his mother, his cooking and so on. I should think he has a grievance against her for this. Certainly in sending him off to study physics they were not intending to bolster his femininity.

There's a distinction to be made in male homosexuality between effeminate homosexuals and perverse homosexuals. The former are very unhappy because they fall in love with masculine men who don't want anything to do with homosexuality; whereas the perverse homosexuals form communities. Freud's description of Leonardo is in the category of the motherly homosexual. You see the same two categories in paedophilia: the maternal and the perverse type.

Sixth recent session

HM: The patient says he's feeling terribly cold, cold in the bones; a sheet of ice is beginning to form over the lagoon.

Participant: Could feeling cold in the bones have to do with his father's metastasis?

DM: Yes, it could.

HM [*resumes*]:

> **Analyst:** Could this also refer to our relationship?
>
> **Patient:** Yes. I can't help laughing; yesterday I was bold and daring whereas today I'm feeling so low.
>
> **Analyst:** Tell me about it.
>
> **Patient:** It's because of a conversation I had with a woman colleague, an old friend, who made me lose all hope as she said no to my suggestion of having a relationship outside of work. I'm very sad.

DM: A brother–sister relationship. She says no; you can see how it follows from this exhibitionist dream.

HM [*resumes*]:

> **Analyst:** What do you think of this colleague's decision?
>
> **Patient:**She has changed because initially she encouraged me and then said no. She wanted no physical contact.
>
> **Analyst:** And what do you think of your own suggestion?
>
> **Patient:** I think it was the right thing; I waited for her, let her have time.

> (He then states that with men of the world, relationships always start with physical contact and then people decide what they want to do.)

DM: First you put your penis in, then you wait to see what happens. Here is more evidence of projective identification with the father's penis that completely misunderstands the way of the world. He thinks you go around with an erection and one woman after another invites you in.

HM [*resumes*]:

> **Analyst:** Then there were two suggestions; one was a relationship off-duty and the other with some prospect of being realised in time. They are not the same thing.
>
> **Patient** (looking surprised): I said if she wanted to be my lover just for two days, that was fine as well.
>
> **Analyst:** Don't you think you're asking her to put up very

high stakes in this relationship whereas you put up none?

Patient: Yes, I knew it was so.

Analyst: Isn't this like coming to analysis to get as much as possible from it? As you put it yesterday: if it works, I'll stay.

Patient: That's right, my idea of analysis is a little like that; I try to take advantage of it. But not from this woman whom I allowed time for and waited.

DM: The trouble is that if you don't take up the projective identification you begin to sound moralising. As soon as you take up the projective identification, you can deal with it as a failure of thought: that he is unable to think about these things when he is being the daddy's penis. Being the daddy's penis means being an irresistible object: that any woman should be thrilled to have a night of love with you, at most two days, Don Giovanni style. Of the two thousand in Spain, none are supposed to regret having Don Giovanni as a lover; it's only when he kills the father of one of them that it gets serious. This is part of the psychology of the shift from the irresistible nipple to the irresistible penis: the infantile view of these part-objects. It would have been more useful to immediately relate it to the previous dream of the wild driving and threatening women's marriages. His red French penis!

HM [*resumes*]:

> **Analyst**: We need to avoid the increasing chilliness in our relationship; I think of the night of that conversation when you expected your mother to side with you against your father; but as this didn't happen you withdrew within yourself, withdrew your feelings, affection, and perhaps geographically too; another part of your personality is still expecting the mother to shift to your side, for instance to stay with you at home and not leave with her husband as she did last Saturday. Something similar has happened in the relationship with the analysis starting with the first summer holidays last year when you realised you were not my only patient, that I'm not unconditionally at your disposal; since then you've withdrawn although you've been coming to the sessions. With the approaching Christmas holidays this anger and withdrawal will surge up again.

DM: This is all very true, but it doesn't quite capture the projective identification with his father's penis: you may just as well go on holiday, get all the women you want, I'm still your penis and so on. Does he know what kind of car you drive?

HM: Living in Venice, I don't need a car! [*Resumes*]:

Patient: Yes, I always react with a withdrawal and try to conceal it. I realise I'm beaten at the end of all relationships.

DM: I think it is true: you have caught him unlike the police who didn't catch him. You have in effect told him that he is treating this woman badly; and in that way you have enacted the policeman-daddy's role; but you haven't quite explained to him how he gets in a state of mind of such arrogance – treating a woman that way who has been his friend for so many years. Because in fact he is not a bad arrogant fellow; this is just a sudden state of mind he has got into – the sequel to running about with a hammer in his hand breaking windows.

HM: I said it seemed to me that the one who gets restrained is the child with the golden thimble put on his penis by his grandmother and aunt, and who turns increasingly violent in his dreams, almost a criminal at night; but the grown-up man in him also learns to listen to and consider others gradually. We'll see if the child can bear being further restrained with the pain and anger the golden thimble inflicts on him.

DM: It's good to bring it back to this material, to the child in him, whose little penis is the sun of the world. I'd forgotten about that. Dangerous creatures these aunts.

It is a very nice way to talk to him. But talking in terms of the child and the adult doesn't quite capture the delusional attitude that has sprung up so suddenly, in his proposal to this woman friend and his amazement that she should refuse him. It's the delusional identification with the father's penis that needs to be clarified; and this only goes halfway to doing that.

I think in going on with him, you mustn't forget the programme of anxieties that were declared in the first dream: fear of water, fear of violence, the inability to be one of the boys, along with the fear of homosexuality. All of those need to be worked on, not just concentrating on his inability to have sexual intercourse. That will come in due time when he is able to relate to a woman in an adult way. But all of these anxieties have to be worked through.

But you are certainly in a very strong position now as a combined object.

The trouble with the way you have talked to him here, which I call moralising, is that if it is listened to as a good father explaining about feminine psychology it is very nice; but it can easily be listened to as teaching him the techniques of seduction. That gets more like a big brother who says 'well the first time you go out you just hold her hand; next time you put your arm around her; the third time you do this ...'. There is plenty of indication that the dream about the wild driving is a projective identification with you as a kind of Don Giovanni daddy. His femininity is strong enough for him to identify with all your women patients whom he will see as falling in love with you, and you with them; but you are very patient with them, you don't have intercourse with them the first year, you wait till the third ... That is the sort of thing you have to be aware of – his bisexuality; his femininity is very strong; his masculinity is just beginning to come into possession of sufficient aggressiveness to be able to penetrate a woman.

It's big progress for just a year and half of analysis.

CHAPTER NINE

A case of transvestism
(1994)

Valeria Mozzon

Petty crime, prostitution, drug trafficking, transvestism, and gang activity are all situations which Meltzer's remarks regarding the following case presentation can elucidate.

Two interesting features emerging from Meltzer's comments need to be stressed here regarding this disquieting clinical material in which the patient touches on both transvestism and homosexual prostitution without completely embracing either; we see the core perverse phantasy on the one side, and egocentric values on the other.

The core perverse phantasy

In his observations Meltzer is following a line of thought that like a thread weaves in and out of different manifestations of perverse phenomena (sexual games, transvestism, homosexuality, prostitution) without losing his direction in their rich array and without mistaking the manifested behaviour for the mental significance of their multiple behavioural forms. The crucial feature of any perversion is sadomasochism. However, Meltzer here makes a further distinction between the many possible variations of sadism (passive seduction, victimising attitude, manipulation, despotism, tyranny, mutilation, etc) and the core phantasy underlying all such manifestations: killing the internal child and the potential creativity of the mother as an extreme act of manic jealousy.

Freud discovered that the phantasy of 'a child being beaten' would often excite perversity; but he couldn't locate where mentally and internally that highly real and powerful phantasy occurred. It was Melanie Klein who in her research located that spot inside the mother's body, which explains why sadistic attack is experienced on a phantasy level as an attack against a potential baby in the womb. In this instance, notes Meltzer, it is the mother's rectum where the imaginary crime is perpetrated. The destructiveness of such a violent phantasy is immense, as is the latent persecution phantasy it generates, as may be deduced from this particular patient's symptoms of anxiety and insomnia.

The delinquent perversion is entirely organised around this core phantasy which destroys what is good and in so doing annihilates creativity.

Egocentricity

At the very beginning of the second session the patient wants to know if the therapist has thought about him. Meltzer does not let this egocentric moment slip by: pointing out that he wants to be sure the therapist's mind is entirely available for himself alone. Later on this egocentric tendency starts manifesting itself more clearly: the patient doesn't distinguish between people, everybody is the same to him, they all fulfil a single role, they exist for and hold on to him and revolve around him; there is neither the recognition of the other as a person nor is there any respect for their feelings. The crucial point, says Meltzer, is A's inability to love, yet his 'eagerness to be the object of others' desire'. Meltzer interprets both masochism and exhibitionist transvestism in relation to the patient's egocentric passivity and their overriding wish to be the object of other people's admiration. It is important to differentiate, as Meltzer does, between the desire to please

– which leaves the person always dissatisfied – and emotional commitment, the essential condition for experiencing a love relationship, free from the feeling of emptiness that requires ever more promiscuous sexual encounters. It is emptiness rather than pleasure which is the driving force, a constant excitement that leaves the patient feeling hollow.

Egocentricity is a subjective state characterised by a world of infantile values which manifests itself in different ways and degrees; it takes other people's unconditional readiness for granted and leads towards the tyrannical need to receive exclusive attention. Only after crossing the threshold of the claustrum can the person enter a depressive state and experience more mature and sophisticated values.

Summary of the first two meetings with Bruno

Bruno seeks my help at the suggestion of his doctor owing to his state of anxiety and sleeping problems. He is 30 years old, tall and slim, with the look of a teenager. He moves slowly with measured gestures, as though trying to avoid causing disturbance.

Bruno left high school in the fourth year, after failing a year, and started working as an errand boy in a company, then got married to a slightly older woman (age 33). The couple married against everybody's advice when Bruno was eighteen, after running away from home. He has been married for twelve years. His son is nine years old. He talks of his wife with gratitude; his marriage, he says, has turned him 'into an adult', gained him his parents' respect, especially his father's, and his wife has given him the impression of 'feeling a man.'

At the beginning of the consultation he says he has problems being with his wife, his son, and particularly his own parents. He mentions physical complaints, such as stiffening of his arm and leg muscles, sweaty palms, and being in a state of panic lest he cannot hide his state of discomfort.

Before getting married he used to live with his parents and his sister, seven years his junior. He enjoyed a good life until the early years of adolescence, then 'something broke' and the conflicts, particularly with his father, started. 'He'd hit me hard, humiliate me, even spat at me once.' He feels deep bitterness toward his father, who is in fact his stepfather; his mother was widowed before Bruno was born and remarried when he turned five. Until that age Bruno lived with and was brought up by his grandparents and his mother's sister: 'I wanted to have a father just like the other children in the kindergarten, and when I finally met my father and we all went to live together I was happy and proud of him.'

Bruno's stepfather is a retired military officer; Bruno talks about how much he admired his stepfather's profession, and recalls the tenderness, attention and love he received from and exchanged with him. It was his stepfather who often looked after him as his mother was in charge of a children's clothes shop and would be away from home for long hours. 'Even when I was ill, it was my stepfather who cared for me, not my mother. I loved him very much and most importantly I felt I was like other children, had a dad, on top of all one with a military uniform.' Bruno has two surnames – his natural father's and his stepfather's, who adopted him so that Bruno's wish to bear 'the same surname as dad's' would come true. Bruno used this second surname alone for years, and shortly before his wedding started also using his birth surname; now he has altered this choice again and uses only his birth surname.

During the first meeting he keeps his hands clasped on his lap, in a rather feminine attitude, speaks in a low voice, and hardly lifts his eyes in my direction.

Donald Meltzer: The first information we have about him brings to the foreground his insecurity in relation to his father's death and the possibility that there could be other men in his mother's life even before her husband's death.

But first we need to put a question: Do we know anything about the cause of Bruno's father's death? Who took care of him after he died?

Valeria Mozzon: His father died of pneumonia. Bruno's mother's parents looked after him: his grandmother and especially his aunt. His father's family wouldn't step in as they had broken up with his mother. Both Bruno and his mother continued using the deceased father's surname. Before marrying another man, his mother often took Bruno to the cemetery to show him his father's tomb, and spoke to him about his father. Bruno recalls these visits as instances of which he could make little sense.

DM: His mother must have encountered difficulties in consolidating in Bruno the concept of his deceased father's existence as a real person. Later on, at five, the figure of the stepfather takes over: a retired military officer who in the child's eyes is certainly a fascinating figure and who somehow seduces him and distances him from his mother.

At this point, though, we need to ask another question: has Bruno got brothers and sisters?

VM: Yes, Bruno has a sister from his mother's second marriage.

DM: I thought it would be so: this helps us understand how, at a certain point, this young boy distanced himself from the maternal figure and came into conflict with her. Apart from his father's death and the fascination his stepfather no doubt had for him, the conflict could have also been generated by the birth of other siblings.

Towards puberty and early adolescence his life story crumbles and falls into a thousand pieces: he's no longer able to continue his studies and with the resulting failure, cuts short his schooling; conflicts arise with his stepfather and the latter treats him brutally. Such a situation little by little turns him into a very quiet, gentle and absolutely non-aggressive boy; he'll then catch the attention of the person who will become his wife (three years older than himself) and who, by marrying him, will become the figure to rescue him from his family environment. Bruno will be intensely attached to her but will remain very passive towards her.

We can already see in such a situation the basic features of a familiar pattern: Bruno will take possession of 'his own' son, distancing him gradually from his wife and setting up conflicts which will result in the couple losing interest in one another and end in their separation.

Bruno's life is dominated by female figures, by his wife in particular. From the point of view of object relations he is in a very unstable state: a situation of instability ruled by jealousy, by constantly coming close to and distancing himself from the object, by a continuous projection of jealousy towards both female and male figures. All this is basically centred on a specific event in Bruno's story: the birth of another baby.

We get the impression of him as a nice boy, with very gentle and even infantile features: this certainly makes him very attractive especially to women, awakening among other things their maternal instinct. We are dealing with someone who arouses in others intense jealousy, possessive feelings, excessive attachment, to which he in turn reacts with projections of equally intense jealousy, used principally as a defence mechanism.

VM: During the second interview Bruno is very restrained; I feel he'd like to be transparent, be there yet at the same time not be seen. His attitude calls to mind the modesty and reserve adolescents assume when talking about themselves.

He strongly needs to throw out what he feels inside.

DM: At this point Bruno is likely to start a seduction process with you – a sort of infantile, gentle seduction.

VM: I have a moment of initial reticence while I ask myself whether I can recall what he'd told me in the previous session …

DM: Here Bruno wants to make sure that the analyst's mind is entirely free and therefore ready to be filled by him alone, by his desire to possess, by his egocentricity. This is the beginning of what may be defined as a 'preformed transference' based on Bruno's attitude to women in his family relations. He uses the same mechanism with you as with his wife to draw you into his world.

Every analysis begins with a degree of preformed transference which needs to be got rid of to avoid acting out in accordance with the patient's scheme of things.

Almost every patient initially approaches the analysis as if he'd like to confirm that the analyst shares his own point of view regarding his problem. Bruno's relationship with the therapist resembles that of a judge rather than that of a simple observer. In the first session we observe a sort of testing of the analyst as the patient tries to convince him he has the same viewpoint and the same suppositions. This is precisely what the analyst must avoid.

VM: The patient then tells me of a violent row he had a few days earlier with his wife after getting home too late without telling her.

Bruno has taken up studying, he now attends a night school for a diploma in surveying. This is why he stays out late every night. His wife believes he has another lover and that he is tired of her; she doesn't understand or accept that he has gone back to his studies; more importantly, she refuses to accept what such a commitment entails. Bruno views the possibility of getting a diploma as a significant opportunity to improve his professional life. He regrets his wife's inability to understand his ambition. His wife's attitude distresses him (he calls her 'mother' by a slip of the tongue) as she is so important in his life. He says he always feels he is on a 'razor's edge' in relation to her. His wife has often threatened to leave him; in fact she did a few years ago, and lived a few months with another young man, but then returned to Bruno. He is deeply worried about such a prospect.

DM: Did this occur before or after the birth of their child?

VM: His wife left when their son was three years old; during this period Bruno and his mother looked after the child.

Bruno is very tense while he expresses his anxiety about this; he wrings his hands, wipes the sweat off his forehead, saying it'd be unbearable to have to go through it again; but he's also aware he cannot always obey his wife's wishes. 'Of course, I owe her a lot, because of her I've become a man, but I can't always arrange things from fear of losing her.'

DM: Now let us look more closely at how this young man's scheme of life functions. His life is full of conflictual situations and resentment of them, and he acts such that he will find someone else to rescue him; he is grateful to this rescuer, yet soon afterwards he lapses into being tyrannised and the mechanism of resentment starts again from which he must be rescued by yet another person. A vicious circle of resentment and rescue is thus set up and these two situations alternate continually. In the midst of all this there will always be a baby, another baby, and naturally another sexual relationship.

Bruno likes presenting himself as a victim, yet he is far cleverer than he would have us believe; in fact he shows he can manipulate others extremely well.

VM: Bruno then talks about the first years of their marriage when no-one existed for him but his wife; she was everything, the centre of his universe, his reason for living; they lived secluded from the rest of the world, a situation which changed after the birth of their son. 'From then on we started having rows; my wife accuses me of neglecting her but this is not the case at all; it could be that I've grown up now and need more room for myself. I cannot live according to her wishes alone even if I do owe her a lot.'

DM: He talks to you about his story as a boy would with his mother.

VM: At the end of the second session he talks about the conflicts between his mother and his wife. 'My mother doesn't like my wife and she was happy when my wife left me, she still thinks I made a mistake by accepting her back. I sometimes think they don't get on with each other because they're so similar; they both have a strong and authoritarian character and both enjoy bending others to their will. I believe they tried to bend each other but both failed.'

His wife, however, has a good relationship with her father-in-law and apparently there is a sort of alliance between the two, at least Bruno thinks so, which radiates a sense of exclusion to others.

I feel at the end of the second session as if he were asking me for reassurance that he would not to be shut out if he did something against my wish. Unlike the first session when he hardly ever looked at me, during the second he keeps peeping at me as if trying to control the situation, perhaps fearing to say something wrong.

DM: Bruno is actually trying to make the therapist enter into his life to play the role of a mother, a new lover, new child, and new father. Each of these roles can be replaced by another at this point in his life. There is nothing certain in his relations, all roles are fanciful and depend on a very fragile equilibrium, whose rationale is entirely egocentric. Bruno states: 'I need room for myself.' The diploma hopes to obtain means precisely this room for himself.

The therapist is asked to ally herself with him in a courageous battle to defend his education, which means she can be a good father, a good mother or a good wife for him; or, she can represent a child for whose sake Bruno is trying to improve himself. It is necessary first to clarify with Bruno the real reasons which make him want to study, which will mean dealing with the irritation this will arouse. What is likely to emerge is the figure of another man whose role is to encourage Bruno to pursue his studies, showing him the economic benefits of his diploma and so on; it will frame a kind of homosexual seduction, just as earlier there was a seductive and fascinating man in the story (the new father) when his mother remarried and had another baby.

The third meeting

Bruno arrives slightly late, just a few minutes; he looks very excited, falls heavily into the armchair, gasping for some time, then breathes normally again. He apologises, saying he had problems at work and feared not making it to the appointment in time. 'It's been a hard week, I was full of anxiety, especially on Wednesday. I felt everyone could read my inside state, that I had become transparent.'

I ask him what they could have read in him and if anything had occurred the day before in particular.

He pauses, lowers his eyes and does not answer.

After a short while and with much embarrassment he starts talking again. 'On Tuesday night something occurred which hadn't in the last two months. I was hoping to have been able to do away with of the tranquillisers the doctor had prescribed, but I couldn't.'

Again he pauses, swallows hard, rubs his hands as though he were searching for words to express himself. 'I don't know how to tell you what happens to me, telling it to you makes me feel very ashamed, but it's this that is my real problem.'

He starts talking again with great difficulty, saying for many years he has been unable to resist the strong impulse to go to the bathroom to put on women's clothes and he experiences great pleasure doing it. 'It's like a ritual, I have to do it, but then I'm inundated with anxiety about it.'

The anxiety, that used to last just a few days, has been torment-ing him daily now for months. He's afraid of being caught by others at night. His wife has suspected nothing so far, although the ritual started a year after they married. Now that the impulse has become far more powerful and irresistible, he has been doing it more often and is ever more afraid of being discovered by his wife. He puts on his mother's and his wife's clothes. He says he has never derived much pleasure from his wife apart from when he gets dressed like a woman, puts on makeup and watches himself in the bathroom mirror, pretending to act like either his mother or his wife. 'It is afterwards that I suffer: I think of what I've done, I think I'm not normal; then that I panic with the fear of being found out.'

He falls silent again and after a brief interval says he is mainly afraid of men who might discover what he does at night. 'On Tuesday my colleagues were looking at me at work, I felt they knew it and were judging me, particularly two of them, an old and a middle-aged one, both my superiors. I've been dreading it ever since I started putting on women's clothes; but at first I could handle it, had no fear, and now I can't help thinking about anything else but being caught. If they find it out, I'll lose everything, my family, my job, and respect; I cannot and do not want this to happen, I can't afford to lose everything …'

He utters these words in a whisper, almost under his breath, as if he feared something else, something really bad and even more dangerous might come out of his mind. For ten minutes he doesn't change position; then lifting his head he looks at me as if wishing to make out if anything has changed; then he looks around at the bookcase, the other empty chair, the pictures and flowers. He seems to be comforted at finding everything in its usual place and I tell him so. A vague smile appears on his lips and he sits more comfortably in the chair.

'It's like coming out of a nightmare; I've never told this to anyone, one can't live alone carrying such a burden.' When he starts talking he is more at ease. 'I'd better tell you all, and get it off my chest. I was eleven when I first discovered I got pleasure from wearing women's clothes. I was playing with a friend in the attic and by chance put on my mother's clothes, which gave me so much pleasure that I had an erection. I didn't know what was happening to me but I felt good. Afterwards I tried to experience the same pleasure by going into my parents' bedroom and putting on my mother's clothes. It was not like the first time, but I managed to get excited and enjoyed it immensely while masturbating.'

He notes that a part of this pleasure of putting on women's clothes and masturbation derives from watching himself in the mirror. This is the erotic pleasure he likes best; at times when making love with his wife he needs to evoke this phantasy of transvestism to get excited. 'When I imagine wearing women's clothes, I'm able to reach orgasm and conclude the intercourse.'

DM: It is very significant that Bruno needs this secret perverse phantasy in order to succeed in having sexual intercourse with his wife. When we work with patients like this, with individuals with sexual perversions that they gradually allow to come to the surface, the problem is that they try to hide the sadomasochistic quality of their form of perversion in whatever way they can. They refer to their problem as though it were simply a matter of polymorphous sexuality (as defined by Freud) and thus they present it in a way that minimises its significance.

It's certainly true that all forms of sexual perversion are polymorphous; it is so because most occur at a pregenital stage and therefore are characterised by all sorts of confusions. The main problem, however, consists in the patient's resistance to disclosing its sadomasochistic nature. Such patients generally seek analyst's help not so much to free themselves of their sadomasochistic perversion but to remedy the negative results such a feature entails; nevertheless the pleasure of such a perversion is too great to wish to get rid of it. They want only to be rid of the symptoms, which are generally depression and persecution. When they seek to hide the sadomasochistic aspect of their perversion they actually try to hide the gravity of the problem, making it appear a subjective or cultural matter dependent on culture and ideas of morality, such as 'even in ancient Greece … in certain cultural circles …'. It is as if their problem were not particularly serious at all, while they succeed in avoiding acknowledging its fundamentally sadomasochistic feature and the resulting vicious circle.

Going back to Bruno's story, we see that his problem is revealed during the third analytic session. Now we know the form the perversion takes; but what has not been spoken about is its hidden sadomasochistic content. And when the analyst attempts to bring this to light there will no doubt be an attack from the patient; she will be accused of behaving just like his mother and wife – of being authoritarian, tyrannical, despotic, and of loading him with too many and too high expectations just as his wife, mother and father did.

As he is a highly intelligent and cunning person, the only possible way to let the innately sadomasochistic aspect of his form of perversion emerge is through dream material. At this point we could simply say that he has serious personality problems and that the only way to try to bring them to light and solve them is through the analysis of his dreams and phantasies.

VM: This is precisely the problem; for at least six months Bruno has referred to no phantasies or dreams. In the last three sessions, however, he has talked about three dreams.

DM: Every perverse person who consults an analyst solely in order to have his symptoms relieved presents serious difficulties with therapy. If he had sought a priest instead of an analyst he could make a full confession of his confusion and express his suffering and anxiety; indeed that is what he is expecting, from the priest and also from the analyst – to be absolved and to enjoy the peace and comfort of absolution.

In the specific case of transvestites the analyst, or similar person, will find himself under gentle pressure from the patient who will do his best to have his problem defined as a question of his personality and sexuality, with features that point to an artistic spirit (no doubt the names of Michelangelo, Leonardo, and of ancient Greek figures will pop up) and therefore as something which need not cause excessive worry. This will continue until material from dreams or phantasy becomes available through which the vicious circle hidden within his perversion can be demonstrated to the patient.

VM: Bruno has now got it off his chest, at least a substantial part of it; his anxiety seems truly diminished at the end of the interview, indeed he looks far less tense as shown by his more relaxed body posture.

I felt I could do nothing but receive what he has brought and so help him modulate the intensity of his anxiety.

We discuss our plan for therapy. As he is economically anything but affluent, we agree to meet the necessary minimum number of sessions – that is just once a week.

Notes on the patient's recent evolution

There have been numerous changes in Bruno's life during these last months. He has concluded his studies, received a diploma, qualified as a surveyor, lost his job and presently is getting financial aid from his parents. He has separated from his wife, who now lives with another man. Bruno sees his son regularly and spends the weekends with him. He is now living in a small flat on his own and is looking for a job to lead an independent life. He wishes to be a physiotherapist.

After separating from his wife his first homosexual encounters have been for payment, with transvestites, 'to understand my own sexuality', as he puts it. The experience has been disappointing. 'I didn't like these encounters because I would have preferred being in their place, they took away my role.'

Through his own friends he has entered the homosexual world and is now looking for partners by putting up ads in *The Babilonia*, a gay paper. He is attracted by men who stir strong feelings in him; but to get into contact with such men he needs to imagine wearing women's clothes or being a woman, as was the case with his wife (and the two short subsequent relationships he had with two other women.) He doesn't accept homosexual couples, feels different from them, and feeling his transvestism puts him in phantasy on a heterosexual level.

He envies the freedom to have many partners yet condemns it. He dreams of having a stable relationship in which he'll play the woman: 'Only in this way can I express my sexuality.' He secretly watches women and their movements; he doesn't accept his male body and would like to be an ephebe with no defined sexuality.

Bruno does not look masculine at all; he has little hair, which is straight and fair, and a lean body. He considers himself very masculine and his body bulky. He has talked of a phantasy he had as a teenager, connected with a comic story about a woman warrior, an amazon with a female body and male strength.

DM: Bruno's case is now evolving rapidly: under the 'protective aura' of the analyst he is now able to make a determining change in his life: he leaves his wife, his work and commits himself to homosexuality. Now it is no longer the anxiety that persecutes him but the terror of women and the state he finds himself in. The dissatisfaction with his body and the impossibility of getting purely female pleasure out of it is growing. He hates his male body so much that he wishes it were transformed into a female one; he seems even ready to undergo an operation, to emasculate himself to attain this pleasure.

VM: So far he has had two brief relationships with men of his age; he has suffered very much as he couldn't let himself go; he longs for the relationship, then becomes tense and blocked because the other is a man like himself. After a relationship he has a strong anxiety (sweating, shaking, tachycardia) which can last from several hours to several days. Of the two relationships he's had with men the one with F meant more to him – a doctor of his own age who for several reasons, such as his tenderness, gentleness and demeanour, resembled his stepfather. They stayed together for three months after which F broke up the relationship abruptly to return to his previous partner. Bruno felt betrayed, abused, abandoned, and for several sessions spat out his anger against F.

In the course of each session Bruno always complains about not knowing where he belongs:

'I can't express my sexuality with the body I have.'

Reflections on the process so far

After the initial sessions I have the feeling Bruno has grown socially but not emotionally; the way he relates is idealised in terms of either 'all' or 'nothing'; I also feel he attributes to me the same superego function that he first did with his mother (who stopped him from having access to his dead father) and then his wife (who got in the way of allowing him 'to be himself'.) His attitude towards me is highly seductive, at times adoring; I clearly feel he wishes to keep me at bay and appease me.

At the beginning of our therapy I didn't inquire into the eroticising aspect of transvestism but rather into the condition of anxiety it brought about. Indeed, in my mind transvestism was an expression of some deeper and far more serious anxiety, which made me worry much more about the patient.

It appeared to me that therapy had to take Bruno closer to his dead father in order to diminish the degree of his anxiety which resulted in the ritual of transvestism. I was experiencing Bruno's erotic phantasy as a manic, delusionary defence mechanism, or rather as a manic attempt to solve his anxiety. I think Bruno was hoping and expecting that his father's persecuting him at night (in his lonely nightmares) would gradually disappear over time and turn into pleasure, rather than guilt.

At first I didn't realise that his manic excitement contained elements of emotional perversion, such as a negative Oedipus complex in relation to his father. All this made me think about the processes of identification with his stepfather, his mother and his mother's sister through me and the therapy. The absence of his real father is likely to have conditioned his deep bond with his mother. His mother dresses her children; this arouses Bruno's jealousy (as happens also in relation to my other patients), and in putting on his mother's clothes he becomes his own mother. Seen in a context of a failure to identify with male features, I thought transvestism was his way of doing it: to safeguard his father's penis. Through transvestism, begun at age eleven, Bruno enacts a phantasy in which he is everything to himself: child–mother, father–son.

In the course of therapy the situation begins gradually to alter: his terror of women begins to emerge; at times I feel I'm like the goddess Shiva in Bruno's eyes, the awful but merciful goddess who lends life through death by receiving human sacrifices. The terror he has of women makes him adore me; he always responds with 'yes, you're right' to whatever I say. On an emotional level he seems to be blocked while I perceive clearly that a process of perversion is going on, something that frightens me. I fear the phantasy of transforming his body from a man's into woman's may pass from an intrapsychic level to a real one. I also worry that the claustrophobic fear, the fear of the object which holds him a prisoner, may lead Bruno to act masochistically.

DM: Let's consider the evolution of his relation with the therapist. If she doesn't give voice to her criticism regarding the new direction Bruno has taken in his life, he takes her silence for mute consent.

However, when she does not concede her usual support or implicit approval, then she is felt to be a woman like all other women, a spoiled object on whom he can vent his envy and critical attitude.

At this point we have the passage where the therapist talks of her own worries regarding Bruno's trouble with his body and how the desire to own a female body may move from an intra-psychic to a real level: that Bruno may decide to undergo an operation to change his physical features.

A recent session

Bruno arrives rather depressed, saying he can't go on like this. 'I can't accept this male body of mine, I don't like it, and I don't enjoy putting on women's clothes any longer. Nor do I want to go to the disco Friday nights with V (a recent boy friend), in women's clothes; he likes it, I don't; for me it's a serious matter. On a rational level I do understand wearing women's clothes helps me because I don't accept I am a homosexual, but on an emotional level that's not what I feel. Ever since I was a boy, actually even as a little boy I'd hide behind the dummies in my mother's shop; they had female bodies.'

I ask him to explain this better as I haven't quite understood it.

'Yes, in my mother's shop there were female dummies with visible breasts and pubis, but without heads; when she wasn't around I had fun putting my head on top of them, having their body, and watching myself in the mirror. The mirror reflected to me the picture of a woman. This was my favourite game, together with dreaming of being a woman warrior.'

Bruno had these phantasies when he was seven or eight.

'I've never felt proud of my body, my penis; on the contrary I felt ashamed of it, I thought it was small.'

He remembers that when he played basketball he'd never take off his clothes in front of the others, nor did he ever have a shower with other players after the training sessions in the gym.

'I don't know what to do, I don't like women, rather I've never felt anything with them; I have felt something in my male relations but only with the fancy of being in women's clothes, better still being a woman; I can't have a relation with a man or a woman just as I am. Still I'd like to have relations with a man but as a woman.'

I say I want to look more closely into his phantasy of being a woman.

At first Bruno rather draws back as if he feared my negative judgement; then he says in the past months he has often found himself wanting to have a female body. 'Transvestism no longer satisfies me, it's not enough. As an adolescent the phantasy of having a vagina instead of a penis did often occur.'

He also recalls not finding any pleasure while looking at naked men or women in pornographic magazines, except for the transvestites; their pictures aroused him often to the point of having an erection. He remembers 'Roberta's Story', a story in instalments in one of the pornographic magazines: 'Roberta was first a man who from childhood felt he wasn't a man, his body was like a prison to him. Once he became an adult he entertained the idea of becoming a woman. He began hormone therapy and his appearance grew increasingly feminine. When he left home at 20, he moved to another city and went around like a woman, he was now Roberta. He became a prostitute, had a house and a partner, all in all a normal life.'

DM: Here we realise that the long process of seducing the therapist is still going on; he perceives her as a 'saviour'. He wants the analyst to express a favourable opinion about taking hormones, a likely surgical operation and all those practices which might help him transform his body to the extent at which he would perceive himself at ease. Bruno does not feel like taking these steps on his own, he needs the support and protection of the therapist.

VM: I asked Bruno what had particularly struck him in the story of Roberta.

DM: The centre of attention is ever more focused on the male genital organ: if we could have access to dream material we'd be able to see Bruno's emerging desire to become a woman; furthermore, this desire is always linked with the phantasy that it is a woman who performs the act of mutilation, unmans and steals his penis. This terror of women is underpinned by the suspicion that all women nurture sadistic feelings and really desire to mutilate the male sexual organ. Equivalent masochism from the female perspective would consist in the phantasy of being raped by a man, resulting in a defensive reaction of attack, mutilation, or even murdering the person seen as the aggressor. All too often, unfortunately, we happen to witness couples with such sadomasochistic mechanisms, whose children then exposed to all the brutality triggered by the state of their parents.

An excellent example of this sort of relationship is given in a Japanese film where an adolescent girl seduces an elderly man who becomes prey to an impelling and furious sexual desire which she arouses in him. The relationship leaves him exhausted and eventually he can only reach orgasm when she appears to strangle him. In this violent story marked by strong sadomasochistic impulses, the end comes with the death of the main character who gets murdered and emasculated by his own lover. Although the entire story is premised on a type of psychosis, the film does represent real life situations, bringing to the foreground genuinely interesting contents.

VM: Bruno recalls that what struck him most in the Roberta story was the transvestism through which he became 'Roberta'; and the meeting with his mother when she visits him in his flat.

I ask him to make this point clearer. Bruno then tells me the rest of the story: 'Roberta at first meant to hide herself, she wrapped a bandage around her breasts so that her mother wouldn't notice him as a woman; but then he changed his mind thinking it wiser for her to know it and let himself be seen as Roberta. What moved me was the moment when the two women hugged one another, when the mother accepted her son as her daughter. That part of the story between the two women was really moving. I often turned to those pages to read them over again. I also enjoyed entertaining my own phantasies on this point; I thought of being Roberto/ Roberta, of having feminine looks, I liked the idea of my mother accepting me as a man/woman. I can say Roberto/ Roberta was one of the heroes of my adolescence.'

I believe Roberta's story, hugging the mother, is a reference to me; Bruno is telling the story for me. Being accepted by his mother and by me might, for Bruno, mean no longer being afraid of a woman's revenge (severed heads, the dummies).

I ask Bruno if he has dreamt recently. He answers he dreams a lot but never remembers his dreams. He then adds he gets up every night at two o'clock precisely to urinate, and feels he has dreamt, without recalling anything. He also informs me that as a child he suffered from bedwetting until the age of ten.

Second recent session

The session starts right away with two dreams, something which excites him. He has dreamt and can finally recall his dream. He offers me the two dreams as precious gifts. He begins by telling me the background of the first dream: 'On Tuesday evening I went to a gay couple's house for dinner; I left their house at 11 pm and was walking home; I was wearing a woman's clothes; a car pulled up and the driver asked if I wanted to get in; I did, making it clear I wouldn't make love, it just didn't suit me and that I'd at most play sexual tricks; we drove off, turned into a side street and after a series of sexual games the driver took me back to where he'd picked me up. Then another car stopped, the man thought I was a woman; when he heard me talk he sped away and I got back home.'

The first dream: *I dreamt of the driver of the first car; I was with him in the car and making love; but I was a woman and he penetrated me and I felt intense pleasure, so intense that I woke up, bathed in sweat, gasping for breath, bewildered but happy.*

I ask Bruno if that man reminds him of something or someone familiar. He says the man was neither young nor old and didn't remind him of any particular person. In the dream, though, he met him at the 'madhouse' on the city walls of the town where Bruno was brought up. He recalls the time when as a little boy he'd ride his bike along the ramparts, particularly interested in the area around the 'madhouse' for he knew that was where homosexuals met. He remembered a tall, fair-haired man everybody said was homosexual and he usually saw him there. The man in the dream vaguely resembled the fair-haired man from his childhood.

Going back to the 'madhouse' leads me to think that Bruno may fear losing his mind, going crazy himself. Wanting to become a woman by transforming his body could be a way to master this fear by means of a reversal: getting emasculated so as not to be emasculated.

The second dream: *He is in a car with his parents and a male friend driving up a road in the mountains and at the end they come to a house which reminds him of his grandmother's house in Sicily.* He then talks with emotion of his Sicilian grandmother, his stepfather's mother, with great warmth and love; she loved him more than her 'real' (blood) grandsons and would fulfil all his wishes. He remembers how she'd hold his face between her hands and shower him with kisses. He used to go to his grandmother every summer with his parents. After a short silence he goes back to his dream: *They all go into the house, Bruno instantly finds himself in a room on the first floor; it's a big spacious room, he is naked and seated on the edge of the bed opposite a wardrobe with a big mirror; his stepfather appears behind him, lays a hand on his shoulder and caresses him; he thinks his stepfather is courting him and he feels ashamed; he gets up instantly and goes for help to his friends, a gay couple on the other side of the room with two single beds. His friends say they can't help him because they need to go out to defaecate; then he goes out of the room to ask for someone else's help, he feels he is suffocating. In the other room there's a woman and he asks her to call the emergency help line or an ambulance to go to hospital. The woman doesn't look like she's understood him, then he starts sobbing and asking her to help him as he is suffocating.*

He wakes feeling short of breath. The first thing he recalls of the dreams is that the woman whose help he seeks is his mother.

I ask him who else he's thought about of the dream and he says he has also thought of me.

'You have been on many occasions a mother to me, helped me not to be afraid. You know, it can't be just a coincidence that I chose you as a therapist. My mother's name is the same as yours; I've never noticed this, now after the dream I realise it.'

His father's courting reminds him of his paternal punishments, his complete change after discovering his transvestism, and the pleasure he enjoyed to the point of having an erection when his father hit him or treated him brutally. He tells me of one particular episode: when his father took him by force to a barber shop to get his hair cropped very short, he had an erection.

DM: Bruno is now discovering his passive oral and anal homosexuality towards his stepfather. What terrifies him though is the idea that his stepfather might castrate him, somehow mutilate him. This is why he seeks his grandmother's and mother's help, he wants to be rescued from the danger of castration. They can rescue him by showering his face with kisses; this shows a way to retrieve and rediscover a relation with the breast, instead of the penis. However, this won't solve Bruno's problems, rather it is part of the scheme of the vicious circle: an ongoing alternation of heterosexual and homosexual attitudes, shifting from infantile to adult states, an ongoing alternation between one object and another – from the desperate need to be rescued, to rediscovering the exciting danger of mutilation, from rescue to betrayal – and so on, without attaining a genuine state of stability or equilibrium. At this point then Bruno will turn to the analyst for help, asking her to rescue him and take her part in the vicious circle we have been observing.

We can see clearly how he projects his feeling of being in the 'grip' of a woman who wants to castrate him, or being victim of a man who wants to castrate him (as in the dream with his stepfather), in his ongoing search for a 'rescue'.

The only way for him to break out of the vicious circle is for him to realise that he is the unconscious victim of his own sadism and that the object of this sadism is his mother's other children. This is the focal point of his sadomasochism: the desire to kill other children.

Now we shall turn to his relationship with the therapist again. At this stage of the transference Bruno urges her to seduce him, to 'shower his face with kisses', to protect him from the homosexual evil. The therapist's position is extremely hazardous; indeed when Bruno 'finds out' (notices) the existence of other patients, other children, the situation will again get out of hand. What is fundamentally important at this stage is the interpretation of the dream material that Bruno has brought into therapy: that he is still a child needs to be brought to light – that he is behaving in the same way as he did in childhood while playing with his mother's dummies and watching himself in the mirror, and that he is still a small child when he immerses himself in anal and genital masturbation.

We are getting ever closer to the crux of the matter: Bruno's incapacity to love, his eagerness for love, the desire to be loved passively, to be the object of desire for others. To him it makes no difference whether his mother, his grandmother or his violent father shower him with kisses; it is this very likelihood that makes Bruno lean towards masochism.

In the dream Bruno finds himself in a room with a homosexual couple, asks them desperately for help but the couple refuse saying they must go and defaecate. Let's take a look at this situation. Who could these two homosexuals be? Who could they represent? They represent nothing else but his buttocks where he turns for help to be rescued. He asks them for permission to lay on his hands (instead of being subject to his stepfather's hand on his shoulders), to let his hands play with them so that he can get excitement. The buttocks say no, they refuse to pleasure him by the touch of his own hands: their proper function is to defaecate.

Third recent session

This session was postponed from Thursday to Friday, at the same time.

Bruno starts with a ten minute silence which doesn't seem to me to be particularly filled with anxiety. Rather he seems to be absorbed by something exact, concrete; at any rate he is relaxed, his body too gives no impression of tension. I perceive he has finally allowed himself to do what he had felt like doing without fearing it.

I ask him what he's thinking about.

'I feel divided: on one side there's my transvestism, on the other my homosexuality, they seem two separate things I cannot bring together. I'm no longer happy with just transvestism, I'd like to have a woman's body so that I can enjoy it. I think I've always wanted to be a woman.'

He remembers his early years when until the age of five he used to sleep with his mother and aunt, and his entire world was made up of women: grandmothers, aunt, his mother and other woman friends of the family whom he used to call 'aunt' or 'grandma' depending on their age. Until the age of nine or ten he preferred playing with dolls, dressed and undressed them and played the little housewife; he had a lot of fun playing these games with his little sister or other girls, always younger than him.

He goes back to the game with dummies. 'It came from inside me, as though it had been natural to me to play with dolls and dummies. As I grew I tried to do all the things expected of other boys; I flattered girls, courted them, made as if I were a lady-killer but I never went out with one single girl. I couldn't go any further than insignificant sexual tricks, I got no excitement, on the contrary I got nervous. What I was good at was kissing girls, I'd learned it well, as a technique, but the kiss meant nothing to me. Still I was flattered by lots of girls and envied by my male peers because of my success. I wanted to be like others, but felt I wasn't like them. When I went to the movies to see a film, unlike other boys, in the love or erotic scenes I identified myself with the actress when the male character kissed her, I shared her feelings. If they made love I enjoyed putting myself in the shoes of the actress. This still happens to me when I watch love scenes, I identify myself with the woman not the man.'

After a pause he talks again.

'I enjoy being flattered, being courted, I enjoy other men's attentions and eyes on me; I did have strong emotions with F – particularly when he looked at me with intense desire, tempted me gently, and when he admired me I felt immense pleasure. It is a pleasure which is perhaps stronger than what I feel when making love. All the preliminaries, the courting, to be wanted by the other are for me highly exciting, making love makes me anxious.'

DM: Here we can observe an attitude typical of transvestites: they are not so much fond of the sexual act itself as of being the object of others' desire and admiration – the dominant feature of exhibitionism.

The point which in my opinion is important to consider is the extreme superficiality of Bruno's feelings. His highest goal is pleasure for himself; he wants to experience pleasure above anything although he doesn't raise the question of how he should earn it; he is not ready to pay the price required to receive the pleasure.

Despite his fitful search for pleasure, Bruno is unable to feel anything because he won't let himself be committed, because there is no emotionality. So he won't prostitute himself nor will he degrade his social position. The main problem there-fore is the lack of commitment, the superficiality of his values; or rather the values applied by Bruno are so infantile that we imagine him as still a young boy wandering around on his bike waiting to be seduced.

VM: Bruno continues: 'After making love with F, opening my eyes and finding myself lying next to a man makes me feel uneasy, it is not natural, it is not normal. I feel I've made a mistake and feel sick.'

He also recalls that this feeling of having made a mistake and being sick started after his father caught him while he was putting on women's clothes. 'I can still feel his eyes on me and his contempt; I believe this is why I feel I've committed an error and feel sick. It cannot be natural for two men to make love. I don't like my male body, aesthetically it isn't beautiful. When I imagine it I never see my male genitals, that remains a very misty area, I'd like to have the body of an adolescent, an androgynous, ambiguous body.'

DM: Here we see additional confusion. All relations that are ambiguous, equivocal and uncertain are a source of excitement for Bruno. His pleasure in confusion emerges here too.

VM: When he says he likes the idea of ambiguity I remind him of the woman warrior cartoon. He says: 'Yes, I used to see myself as the woman warrior too, she was beautiful and seductive as a woman and strong as a man; she was unbeatable, she'd punish the bossy and defend the weak.'

I point out that the woman warrior is the picture of a beautiful woman who does not simply destroy but also helps and protects others.

DM: We can see that Bruno hasn't yet formed the concept of desire and admiration, but transforms these feelings into submission, fear etc. What is striking again is his great immaturity which, together with his passivity, allows the domination of not so much the aspects of his perversion and sadomasochism but rather of his incapacity to experience desire and draw pleasure from a love relationship. Bruno is left with a void which can be filled with nothing except sexual contact, constant excitement, and physical pleasure. The logical consequence will be that in order to raise the degree of excitement to its highest level, Bruno (like the character in the film I referred to) will be left with no alternative but to engage in sadomasochistic practices.

VM: Bruno listens to me in silence. Then he says: 'Yes, what you're saying reminds me that I've always felt a woman to be a threat. As a child I was very afraid of my mother and I still am; when she gets angry, she becomes furious. Last summer she threw a flower pot at me. My mother used to resemble the woman warrior in that she too was beautiful and seductive-looking, but she didn't behave like her. I remember my stepfather as a gentle, affectionate man; I don't have tender memories of my mother. My wife is also like my mother, strong and beautiful, but I am in awe of her as I explained before because if I didn't do everything she said she'd threaten to leave me.'

He remembers a dream he had two months earlier and that he'd forgotten: '*I was in a spacious place, like a church with no furniture, the light filtered through the vast windows. I was lying on the floor and next to me there was a not altogether young but very beautiful woman. She was wearing a black chemise, had a beautiful body. She was caressing me and I her, I wanted to make love to her but when I drew myself gently towards her she took out a dagger and tried to kill me. I got scared, freed myself from her embrace and ran away without looking back, afraid of finding her at my shoulders. I remember waking gasping for breath.*'

I ask Bruno who that woman reminds him of.

'All women, in particular my mother.'

I point out how this dream has actually brought us back to the last session and the things we observed together. When I ask him when he had the dream he says he can't remember, perhaps a couple of months ago; he pauses, keeps silent for a while and as though it's suddenly entered his head, says: 'Now I remember, it happened when you postponed the session and we didn't meet for ten days – yes, at the end of September, I'm quite sure.'

DM: Here we should stress a highly significant feature in terms of the analysis: Bruno experiences his disappointment as a blow from the analyst, a sort of betrayal, an act of sadism. It is important to note that Bruno experiences any suffering as a sadistic attack from someone else, and no doubt as something that cannot be forgiven.

VM: I tell Bruno that the woman in his dream could be me in that I first welcome him, flatter him, but then abandon and kill him.

Bruno stays silent, though not a grave silence, and then says: 'Yes, it might be; I too thought it could be you but didn't have the courage to say so, I thought you'd be angry.'

I feel this is the first time Bruno has ever spoken freely to me, without the fear of making me angry, without his usual demeanour of a good, obedient child.

DM: The analysis has now reached a stage where the analyst has increasingly often the opportunity to explore the transference with her patient; consequently, she can look not only at events, phantasies or dreams, but also concentrate on and analyse the transference.

Let us take, for example, the patient's reaction to the postponed session. We realise that Bruno's preoccupations do not allow him to imagine the reasons that might have led the therapist to change the date of the session and hence make him worry about her; on the contrary he has a dream in which the analyst emerges as the person who betrays and attacks him with a dagger. His strongest feeling is of overriding disappointment.

This material can now be analysed to demonstrate to Bruno how egocentric he is and how he feels anxious only about himself. He is not able to feel interest, preoccupation or anxiety for others, for instance the problems that might have caused the therapist to postpone the session. If we examine and describe the transference it is possible to show Bruno the extent to which he is egocentric and superficial, and this method is certainly likely to have more weight than a lecture or sermon from the analyst.

Let us now turn our attention to the beginning of this patient's analysis and its evolution throughout the year. Despite his assertions, he came not wanting to be 'cured' but to seek approval for what he had already decided. What he needed was emotional backing to allow him to cope with the import of his decision to be a declared transvestite and homosexual. He sought the same protection from the analyst as from a guardian angel. As this reveals the way he uses the therapist, it would a good opportunity to look into the transference material and demonstrate to the patient how he conducts his relationships.

The analyst deserves praise as she has been able to arrive at truly significant results for her patient within a year of therapy.

This case reminds me of a similar one where a homosexual patient of mine was able to attain similar results only after a good five years into therapy. Admittedly the patient I'm talking of was 54 years old, and age is certainly a hindering factor in making progress against perversion in an analysis. In Bruno's case, by contrast, age plays a helpful role; it would have been even better if someone had noticed his state sooner and taken him to an analyst as he roamed around on his bike along the city walls.

Nonetheless cases where transvestites are children are by no means easy to deal with, for they also have a strong resistance and act this out in the sessions. But their fluid and malleable character means that the therapy has a higher chance of success than with adult transvestites. We need to bear in mind that although Bruno is 30, he is still an adolescent. My patient is like him but more crystallised. Another difference between these two cases concerns their economic means: while Bruno may be pushed to prostitute himself to make ends meet, my patient is affluent and often it is he who pays another man for sex.

One thing that makes me wonder in Bruno's case is that he is not able to appreciate the beauty of a man's body and is instead attracted entirely by the genital organs. I suppose what accounts for this is the fact that the object is still seen only as a part-object because he is still at a not fully defined stage of homosexuality. If I may make a prediction I'd say if he enters deeply into the analytic transference, Bruno will stay there for quite a long time.

CHAPTER TEN

A boy with a gentle heart: inside and outside the father's head
(1994)

Rodolfo Picciulin

I receive a message on my telephone answering machine: 'This is Mr S speaking. I'd like an appointment with the doctor' (and leaves his phone number). It's a strong yet soft voice with a peremptory tone; I imagine it belongs to a man of between 45 and 50 years of age). When I call back to arrange an appointment the person tells me he has got my name from his doctor, but says nothing about his reason for seeking a consultation and I make no inquiries.

First consultation with Luca

Mr S comes to the first appointment in the company of a sixteen or seventeen-year-old boy. I ask them to take a seat in the big room where I do group therapy and Mr S starts talking. He's a big, robust man with a glowing complexion. The boy sitting next to him is long-limbed and neat, and looks intelligent. The man begins by saying he's come because of something that happened two years ago and that it has to do with him but he prefers his son to talk about it. He's thought it worth coming to me despite the long period of time that has intervened. At the time they had been advised to have some family therapy but later believed it wasn't necessary to pursue the idea. Mr S says it's his son's problem, which is why he's brought him to me. Finally I grasp who the youngster is sitting next to him.

At that point the boy introduces himself, stating he agrees with what his father has said so far. I ask him whether he himself wishes to add anything else but he answers no, preferring to talk alone with me. I invite him in to the consulting room which is adjacent. At that point I am thinking I've made a blunder: I'd taken the father to be the patient, instead it's his son. Well … we'll see.

Luca is a sixteen-year-old boy in his third year at high school (the classical *liceo* he tells me later). He seems very open, polite, and speaks very much to the point. He sits down on a chair and tells me how he agreed with his father's idea of coming to me, partly to go along with his father's wishes and partly out of curiosity. (His explanation has a very positive effect on me.) He says he's got over the problem that his father referred to and that lay behind his coming here, although it's not at all very clear as yet. (Now I've grown rather impatient and wish to hear the real reason.) He talks about his desire to kill himself, or rather ideas of that sort that he entertained in the past. He notes how those ideas had to do with certain nihilistic principles that he held, ethical motives, and logical thinking. These had pushed him to think of committing suicide. Wishing to kill himself has been his constant thought. He tells me one of the major obstacles to his very likely suicide are his parents, for they'd suffer immensely. He's very closely tied to them and fears neither his father nor his mother could stand such a violent action of his. For this reason he thought that in order to achieve his desire he'd first have to kill his parents and afterwards himself.

Then he tells me what happened in January two years previously when he was fourteen years old. He had been getting ready and thinking how to 'do it'; then one day he stood in wait for his father to come back home and on his arrival attacked him with a hammer, giving him six or seven blows on the head. His father was wounded but managed to stop him. His father, bleeding, called for help to his wife; the two hid his wounds, wiped off traces of blood and decided to keep it a secret. After the assault Luca was a little confused. He says he wept as he hugged his mother; then he went down to the cellar with his father. They thought they'd make up a false accident to account for his father's wounds (say a pile of logs suddenly landed on his father's head). Only a few days later did Mr S turn to a psychiatrist friend who suggested they begin a family therapy. But eventually they decided not to.

I ask Luca what he thinks about what happened and what his parents think.

'From then on my father hasn't said a word to me about it. When we argue, on several occasions he has reproached me for attacking him; my mother hasn't spoken about it again and she doesn't want to. It's a taboo. To her it's as if it hadn't taken place at all. But I, when I think about it, don't know …it was something I had to do to be logical about my ideas.'

I ask him what he thinks today of what happened. He remembers that as his father was being hit with the hammer he cried something like: 'What have I done? What have I done to you? What have you done?' When his mother came Luca stopped hitting and ran to her, hugged her and cried; then he ran into his own bedroom with the hammer and the gun was on his bed.

'Gun? What gun?' I ask.

'Ah, well, yes, my father's gun. I'd taken it away from him to …'

I am shocked and instinctively say: 'You haven't told me about this. Why didn't you use the gun?'

He says: 'It would have been too loud and would have attracted the neighbours.' (I realise I'm too 'hooked on the events' and wonder to what extent it could be showing off, provocation or something else …).

'My idea,' says Luca, 'was to kill first my father, then my mother and then commit suicide. I'd have used the gun in the end.' He says his father has a licence to carry a gun; when he'd bought it from a gun shop in his home town, Luca was with him and several times went with him to buy bullets. He recalls once his father fired the gun in the cellar, which terrified all the neighbours.

Luca says he knew where his father kept the gun and that he'd go and have a look at it every so often. He also says he has a knife collection, lots of knives although one of his cousins has a far 'richer' collection than he.

Donald Meltzer: Is this the first time he's mentioned his cousin?

Rodolfo Picciulin: Yes.

Then I ask him if he can recall how he nursed the idea of rebelling against his parents. Luca puts it in the autumn of 1991, when he was fourteen, after he'd seen the film *The Doors* with Jim Morrison. The film and the character had struck him immensely; it had left him bewildered and baffled. He'd always liked the macabre. At elementary school on several occasions he'd shocked his teacher with particularly macabre, horror-filled stories. He says Jim Morrison is possessed by a native Indian spirit that entered him at an accident he witnessed when many Indians lost their lives; after that he (Morrison) became Indian himself. That was when Luca started to think about wanting to die, and did what he actually did.

He tells me little more about himself, adding that he likes writing poetry and stories.

DM: The idea behind the killing and the suicide in this case means transforming himself into someone else, for instance Jim Morrison who becomes an Indian. This is an example of projective identification even if brought about in a violent manner: he attacks his father with hammer blows in order to become the father himself.

In line with the rules of what we might call psychic reality, the degree of mental disturbance in projective identification is proportional to the degree of violence involved in the mechanism. So if you hit someone, say with a rake, from a psychic and mental view there'd be eventually less harm than using a pistol.

RP: He then tells me two of his stories in detail. I shall relate one which begins: 'A man was kept in a box from the day he was born; he's already in his 40s or 50s. He remembers nothing about his childhood because at one stage he gets lost in a vicious circle (he thought that he thought that he thought …).'

DM: As is the case with most of us, a particularly dangerous vicious circle.

RP: 'When he comes out of the vicious circle he is 20 or 30; he is at a research centre being experimented upon; he is fed through a pipe which a nurse fills with food; he grows in this box, kept in a foetal position. When he eventually comes out, he's misshapen, dirty and disfigured after all those years spent tightly enclosed in a box.'

Luca's parents

Luca is an only child. His father teaches literary subjects and his mother works in public administration. I had one consultation with Luca's parents and three meetings with Luca before starting therapy. I suggested Luca come twice a week but later he said he had a lot of work at school so we arranged to have one session a week until June and afterwards increase this to two.

At the consultation with the parents I related what had emerged from the initial meetings with Luca, taking into consideration the fact that the patient is underage; and I would like to hear the parents' side of the story. In retrospect I should say the meeting didn't help me much, other than to strengthen the impression I had formed of his father as a very intrusive man who tends to speak on Luca's behalf and insert himself in his place. I heard them talk to one another as if they were brothers, equals.

DM: Is this something you're saying to yourself or to them?

RP: This what I think to myself.

DM: What does his father do?

RP: He's a teacher at a secondary school and his mother is a state employee.

DM: Has the gun got anything to do with his job?

RP: No, I suppose he might use it for hunting.

DM: Did you find out why they had waited so long before consulting you?

RP: No. Some minor event occurred which made them eventually consult me: while talking to friends on the phone the boy mentioned smoking dope. His dad was alarmed and thought of consulting a therapist. His father was upset when I asked to meet both parents (I think they don't have much respect for our kind of work) and got even more upset when I openly asked why he didn't get rid of the gun after what had happened.

Luca's parents don't seem to communicate openly and directly between themselves, nor do they share the same views. The mother is very reserved and stands to the side. She never intervenes unless I ask her opinion. She looks much younger than her husband and appears to withdraw herself from the discussion, saying that is something 'the two men' should deal with 'between themselves'. Later on with much fear and intense feeling she told me what happened that day and at the end burst into tears.

Beginning therapy

The initial sessions are quite cold and too intellectualised. I have the impression Luca wishes to show off all his 'knowledge' (he speaks like a book). He talks so hurriedly that I find it difficult to find room to say something. It looks like I need to take time.

I ask Luca if he remembers anything in particular. He replies he's got a lot to tell me. When he was a child he'd often get angry – 'I was violent, I'd lose my temper, I'd take it out on spiders and pull their legs.' At elementary school he'd try to terrify his mates with awkward demonstrations, like making the sign of the cross. He recalls his teacher once told his parents to see a psychiatrist. He also recalls sleeping with his head under the pillow. He used to adore characters like magicians, 'riders of the dark', sinister figures. He dreamt of being 'an enemy worthy of respect', a sort of untouchable figure like Dracula whom intelligent people would admire. He mentions Dorian Gray, whose very sight inspired 'fear and admiration'. He imagined that when grownup he'd have no family and would live in a small flat or hotel room and spend his days wandering around aimlessly.

He couldn't imagine having children of his own. He says: 'I've always dreamt I'd live alone, by myself, probably in a big city; perhaps work as a detective as in Marlowe's films, or alone in some castle somewhere such as Bavaria surrounded by a herd

of attendants like Dracula – he's always been a hero to me, a
fascinating character. In my third or fourth year at elementary
school I was really interested in minerals and dreamt of being
a geologist when I grew up. Then I saw films that impressed
me and made me want to do something important like being a
journalist or a writer. Now when I think of the basement room
I remember wanting to be a designer; I adore maps, like the
maps of the Military Geographic Institute – perhaps so as to
keep everything under control.'

Then he talks about some dreams. The first was from some
time ago:

'I remember a dream from a long time ago. *As I was going
downstairs to the kitchen to get something to drink there was a doll
sitting on a step with a fork in its hand. I was terrified; 'Keep quiet'
said my mother, 'you might wake it up.' I remember I had a doll as
a child, a small one; it had feet but I can't remember if it had legs
too; it was made of black wool, its face looked somehow human,
the fork was like a devil's, made of wool; it must have suffered
from the heat in summer.* There were other dreams too. One
time in bed I noticed something was moving on the wall, it
had six legs, six yellow-black legs; I was stunned, couldn't move
– couldn't even reach out to switch on the light. I thought of
what I did in the summer time when I'd capture yellow-green
spiders and put them in a transparent box (used for shirts), I
had one entirely filled with spiders …'.

I wondered whether in talking about the shame and panic
that he felt Luca was also referring to his dead grandmother.

DM: We see that the patient is now telling us the story of
his life. Normally a quite precise and detailed picture of the
patient's life story is given. This story (more or less similar to
the one that actually happened) is what he himself has made
up about his life and it helps to cover confusions, forgotten
fragments and other things. On the whole we are dealing here
with a boy in puberty. When we listen to the stories boys tell in
puberty or adolescence, they all give the impression of borderline psychotics their childhood reactions, even if this may not
necessarily be the case. It is a little like a description of latency
from the perspective of adolescence: latency being experienced

as a claustrophobic period, as represented clearly by the box with the man inside. As a result, puberty and adolescence are the equivalent of leaving, coming out of this claustrophobic state.

In this particular case, it also has to do with intruding into the object so that this person becomes even more psychotic, more seriously borderline than before. What surprises us is the fact that his violence has been expressed in such a real way, namely by attacking his father. For he is essentially a fairly good and calm boy. His violence, his conflicts could have been imagined instead of being externalised as in fact took place.

Generally we learn little from the stories told by patients of his age at the beginning of analysis, of consultation. These stories need to be regarded as fictional tales, intended to produce an effect on the analyst; in this case the story aims at evoking the suspicion that there are strongly perverse tendencies fixed at an orally sadistic level. This gives us a picture of an Oedipal family situation where the mother presides over a ferocious, lethal battle between a bull and a bullock; she is terrified by what will ensue and regards herself as the prize of this mortal fight, which makes us think of Freud's description of the primal scene that is the foundation of the Oedipus complex.

With youngsters in this age group, the analysis begins with a preformed transference based on the story that best represents their mood at that moment. We will see that this preformed transference will change into a genuine transference relationship which will emerge simply because the analyst refuses to play the role assigned to him in the preformed transference.

In this case the preformed transference consists in containing and preventing the potential murder the youngster may commit, even though we do note that here the analyst isn't so impressed by the homicidal aggression of the boy as by the father's interest in arms and weapons, which is reflected in his son's passion for a knife collection, marking his anxiety about coming under attack and therefore his need for self-defence.

You're going to talk about a session in May; when did Luca start analysis?

RP: At the end of February. In early March we had the first interview, then the Easter holidays came up.

DM: Did the analysis then start after the Easter break?
RP: Yes.

Two months into therapy

In the session of 2nd May Luca tells me of his grandmother's unexpected death:

'Last week my grandmother died (my father's mother). My grandfather (my mother's father) had died two months earlier. There was a storm in the family: my grandmother had a stroke, fell down and died (I was at school and they called me). There were dramatic reactions; I didn't cry although this was the grandmother I went to spend my summer holidays with. She was very good. Instead I felt embarrassed because my father was crying. My father was very attached to my grandmother (although she considered him the black sheep of the family); he'd take her shopping in town. Someone has gone missing. I was feeling not grief but embarrassment for my father and I didn't know what to do. When I came back from school my mother was crying, my father was at the opposite end of the room; I hugged my mother and she said 'Go to your father.' I didn't know what to do. The day before we'd argued. Even later, talking about the funeral, all the relatives …what a mess. I had self-control, but Dad broke down, so did my mother.'

Luca says earnestly: 'Oh, wish I could have cried! But I couldn't, I felt bad, I wish I had cried …The next day things got better; my father was putting together the documents for inheritance matters. My nerves were still on edge. I felt everyone's eyes were on me at the funeral; I didn't want to look at my father and the other relatives as they lowered the coffin. My grandmother who was always very pale was now whiter than the silk lining; I enjoy horrible things so long as it's in a book or a film; but there … I had a dream, a dream that partly repeats itself. *I was in the classroom at school. My art history teacher was asking me something, it was an oral exam. The book was open on the desk as usually happens but I couldn't read the text before me. It was like when you wake up in the middle of the night and are in a drowsy state. I couldn't open my eyes; it was as if I was blinded by a light before me, like when you press your eyes with your fingers (something I do quite often). I felt dismay; I didn't know what to do, how to behave; I felt alarmed.*

'I had the dream on Tuesday, the same day my grandmother died.'

Luca gave his associations to the dream. He said he was not good at history of art, and knew little about it; they did an hour a week; the teacher came in, gave the lesson, went out. He has had to put off his oral exam several times. 'I've put it off again and again. I remember in the dream: it was Etruscan art, a black statue, a picture of a lion's head with something on its back' (he means the chimera: in Greek-Roman mythology this is a lion with a goat's head coming out of its back and a serpent-like tail). 'I am conscious of others' presence and I can't read, I can't understand the subject; I am running away from something.'

He then remembers a dream he had five or six months earlier: '*Someone, some boy or boys wanted to kick me, I was in a great panic. I didn't know where I was, I was lost, disoriented, carrying something on my shoulders.* I thought of the recent sessions, as if I had to comply with it and was afraid of coming into conflict with you. When I don't know what to say I'm filled with dismay, I think I should not be dumb before someone, the silence is not productive. As a matter of fact I've had feelings I can't even define – panic, shame; I'm angry, I lock myself up. I wish I could be more spontaneous … I wish I were …but can't.'

DM: He's a very interesting boy, and has a strong observational capacity: for example he knows and understands that speaking, words, are a defence for him, to keep away the persecutors and defend himself from a sense of claustrophobia. When words fail him, then he falls into a state of panic from confusion. He is a boy who has often thought about death and persecution, but we see that the moment he comes face to face with the true reality of his grandmother's death, he falls into a state of confusion similar to the moment when words fail him.

On the one hand there is the area of thoughts, ideas, fantasies of death, which remain at the level of fantasy and are not acted out; on the other is the real world, the world of projective iden-tification where action takes place.

In line with the preformed transference, we see the patient now feels the analyst is about to persecute him, and speaking will enable him to keep the persecutor at a distance.

RP: Until June we continue the analysis with one session a week. The material is abstract and emotionally distanced even though the patient comes to the appointments regularly and always on time.

Once the school year is over (Luca has to repeat two subjects in the autumn) we start meeting twice weekly, even though there is just a short time till the summer holidays, and we resume the sessions in September. As the general atmosphere gets warmer, Luca tells me about his journey to Rome with a group of friends from Rifondazione Comunista (a left-wing party in parliament of which he is a member) and about what he is doing at school.

I shall present some dreams that Luca brought in the autumn.

First dream

The session before the first dream, which occurred at the end of September, Luca told me he had failed to do something he had promised his friend J. The friend had waited for him at the offices of the Rifondazione party where Luca had said he would meet him, but instead he had gone somewhere else with other friends. He added he felt really guilty. He dreamed: '*Last night I went to bed with my mind at ease although I hadn't yet digested the situation with J. I thought it was over… I wanted to kill myself, considering everything that had gone wrong – J, my school performance, I felt cut off from my friends – the same state I was in three years ago. The decision was final: I only needed to put it into practice. In the dream I did what I'd done on that afternoon two years ago: I went into the basement and I took the pistol. In the room I meant to aim it at my temple with the same degree of intensity.* I'd never dreamed of killing myself, it's an abnormal dream. I immediately feared regressing, not facing the situation, and seeking shelter only in the thought of death. The strange thing is that I went from a state of anxiety to one in which the idea of killing myself flashed like lightning. Perhaps all this has to do with having read some old poems (from that time) which left me a little saddened; I experienced it again through poems and a short tale referring to that afternoon.'

DM: If we go back to what happened, his attempt to kill his father and the plan to kill first his father, then his mother and then himself, this last gesture of shooting himself means waking up, rousing himself out of this state of projective identification, as happens in his dream.

In his description of what happened with his friend J, we can see a typical adolescent pubertal conflict: it's the conflict the teenager experiences between the group and individuality. On the one hand there's the desire to be a group member, to be nearly anonymous, disguised within the group, and this has to do with projective identification; on the other hand there's the desire for intimacy, an intimate relationship between two persons. If one of these desires overrules the other this conflict emerges and results in a feeling of guilt which concludes with: 'Judge me – true, I deserve to be punished.'

For teenagers still in the latency period, this conflict of feeling split between being a group member and intimacy with another individual is not yet substantial, because the group is not seen as essentially delinquent, and moreover the relationship with parents is still quite simple, based on obedience, respect, a sort of non-conflictual loyalty. The contrast is heightened for teenagers on entry to puberty, which is why the peer group comes to be regarded as delinquent by the parents, as it gets linked with problems like sex, politics, drugs for instance.

The same conflict exists in the analytic transference, which contrasts with the need for loyalty, faithfulness towards the group (be it the school or the communist party, etc). Then it also concerns how to spend one's time, more with the group or more with the intimate relationship. Regarding the question asked earlier, about whether Luca's murderousness could be acted within the analysis also, in my view there is no danger of this since we can see he is an intellectual boy who ruminates and ponders in a circular manner (almost in a vicious circle within his own thoughts) rather than a boy of action. We note that his main worry consists in being consistent with his own ideas, his own ethical principles, as he put it; in the transference it stays on this intellectual level. This danger existed principally in the relationship with his parents where we note there is not much communication, much dialogue, and instead the conflict gets transformed into violent action. The fact that the analyst lets him speak about his fantasies is a sort of relief valve which is translated onto the level of intellectual expression instead of action. The only danger might be the interruption of the analysis if and when it comes to interfere with his group life, should questions of loyalty towards the group emerge; in such an event you need to be flexible so as to try to make him come to the sessions.

The boy is worried about being stuck in a vicious circle, that is not being able to leave his worries which persecute him one after the other in a sort of circular movement. We note that he says: 'Right, I'll kill myself but this could cause sorrow for my parents – so I'll kill them first and then commit suicide.' When he attempted to kill his father he believed a single hammer blow would be enough to kill him, as when butchering an animal, intending not to make him suffer – almost a benign, gentle act on his part; this is where his gentleness comes into conflict with his anxiety, with the desire to free himself from such torment-ing thoughts. Finding himself trapped in a circular movement and looking for a way out, a perfect solution to both problems becomes an obsessive question. I think of the case of a patient of mine who wanted to kill her husband by hitting him on the nape of the neck just once with a rolling pin.

As regards the question raised about the potential danger to other patients, well, on the whole such a danger may be excluded. It exists only in paranoid patients who are in thrall to the grandi-ose part of their own personality, the part that gives orders which are then carried out. A paranoid patient has a sort of private reli-gious system of his own, equivalent to (say) a homicidal puritan whose beliefs take the shape of eliminating the world's wicked-ness by killing all those who are in his view malicious.

In this case, the boy's grandiosity hasn't reached any special articulation: we understand he just wishes to become famous, rich, a journalist, a poet or the like. The sole fear regards his not turning into the black sheep of the family like his father. It is not in fact clear to me why his father is regarded as one.

First dream

Some six weeks later, at the beginning of November, Luca brought the following dream: *'It was my birthday and my parents gave me as a gift a prostitute to spend the night with. At first, she looked good and well-proportioned, although I didn't really like her face.* (Her face reminded me of a girl I know who has a face like a monkey's and another one with a face like a she-dog. They are both girlfriends of two friends of mine.) *It was my father and my mother who brought the prostitute home. Three other friends of mine were there too. Instead of taking her to my bedroom, I took her into the dressing room.'* (This is where Lucas does his homework while his mother does the ironing or darning and sewing.) *'It's a rather small room, without a bed. My friends were waiting outside. I started kissing and touching the girl … but halfway someone called me and I left the room. Then I went in again. This happened three or four times. I heard my mother tell my friends outside to leave me alone – she had given me practical advice on how to do it. I grabbed the girl and pulled away from her pubis a sort of a reproduction of the vagina that was blocked with two seals in the shape of an X. It was like removing a plastic sheet, a 10 x 10 cm size sheet. I removed the membrane and penetrated her, and the girl stripped of her membrane looked at me wonderingly, perplexed, and asked: "Did you like it?"'*

His associations were: 'I thought of many things. Of a school friend (older than me and who has a group of neo-Nazi-dressing friends) whose friends had given a prostitute as a birthday gift: a wild bunch, it was his first time. Then there's the wardrobe. It's more exciting in the wardrobe. The wardrobe takes up half the room, which has the ironing board, drying rack, and little free room left: just a strip of fitted carpet. Perhaps I imagined I could do it on the floor. I don't know what to make of leaving and re-entering the room continually but it was as if there was a big party going on in the house and people kept coming to ask me things like: where are the towels, where is the bathroom, the bins … I was surprised by the film-vagina stuck onto her. Now I remember my mother might have come in to help me remove the film – and believe this prostitute looked like a classmate of my friend J whom I always found attractive and I hate her because she feels superior and doesn't yield easily.'

RP: I think the difficulty with J (whom he's very attached to) made Luca revisit and live through again what had occurred a couple of years ago.

I interpret it saying he may have preferred to lose everything (by killing himself) rather than sorting out the conflict between his desire to stay in other friends' company and the promise he'd made to meet J. In the second dream something similar occurs: here it's his parents who provide him with the prostitute-therapist to keep him away from women outside the house.

DM: An excellent interpretation; indeed it perfectly captures the conflict the young boy is experiencing – the conflict between the group on one side and the intimate relationship with a friend on the other, that is hetero and homosexual relationships, the conflict between following the parents' values and being attracted to delinquent ones such as the group of neo-Nazis. On his part there's the effort to find a single solution for everything, a panacea to suit all simultaneously. And again the confusion, this confused mental state as represented by all these characters in the dream who ask him for something. This also stands for his uncertainty regarding the sexual act and its significance.

Third dream

RP: The (following) dream occurred in early November, a few days before Luca's journey to Rome on the occasion of a massive trade union demonstration. He told me nothing about his intention to take part in the demonstration. I came to know about it only afterwards during the session when he talked about the difficulties of this 'first journey', his various moods when discovering 'solitude' (despite being with the Rifondazione group) in a big city in the midst of a demonstration with a million and a half participants. He spent two sleepless nights in the coach with his eyes wide open in fear. He later talked about his terror of getting lost in the demonstration; it was the first time he had the experience of being away from home. I believe joining the

Rifondazione group was important as an opportunity to experiment with something unknown, unfamiliar.

'I dreamt my parents paid for a prostitute for me. I come home with a girl friend, M. My parents, my father in particular, warned me that a prostitute was expected because it was high time I did it. I'm ashamed of having to do it with a prostitute. The doorbell rings. A woman of a certain age (55–60) walks in. Her face looks like that of a woman I met a while ago: a leftwing woman from Rifondazione Comunista who ran a shop selling pins and jewellery and wore heavy makeup. I used to discuss books with her; her shop, Black Moons, was closed down. The prostitute looks like that woman — repulsive yet with a maternal attitude. We go into my parents' bedroom. I have to have an erection, I must, we do it thoroughly. She didn't interfere with me — she made me understand what I had to do until I had an erection. I penetrated her — no problem. Well, perhaps there was some, my revulsion. I went into the bathroom to wash myself. When I went downstairs my parents and my girl friend M were there. The woman remarked on my performance: "He's got difficulties, it doesn't come easy." A critical remark in front of M and my parents.'

Luca's associations to the dream are: 'I think I went a bit further in this dream than in the previous one (the one with the film), besides I was in a queen size bed. I was surprised by my parents' judgement over my performance, they know this woman. I doubt if I described her appearance correctly, perhaps her face was ruined; she treated me like a mother although she did it to get paid. Moreover, she wasn't that old, I ventured to say 55 or 60 because I was afraid to get near your age (the therapist's).

Luca feels he needs to 'get moving' because he's got the impression that if he doesn't do it now, then girls won't be willing to do it with him when he really wants to. Then he adds he may be afraid of whether when the moment comes he'll be fit and succeed in doing it.

DM: This is the essence of the pubertal boy: constantly waiting to be urged on and invited to perform the sexual act, and afraid that when the call comes he will fail to perform.

Session of November 21st

After this, during the session of November 21st, Luca tells me: 'Between yesterday and today I've felt intensely lonely. Saturday night wasn't anything special. I did absolutely nothing – had no minor fun either. Saturday night should be the big day – if I feel like it. I've always done exceptional things on Saturday nights. On Sunday I buried myself in books. I didn't even try to avoid others; I felt useless. All this because J was away.'

DM: Here we notice the beginning of transference, with the experience of separation brought on by the weekend: to such a degree that he let pass the occasion to do something on Saturday night, which is when a sexual encounter could take place. Instead he feels lonely, no longer a special person, does nothing special; and when he says 'On Sunday I buried myself in books and did nothing to avoid others' he actually means 'It's the others who avoided me, I felt useless because J wasn't there.'

Over the weekend Luca sizes himself up, in the absence of J (the therapist). He'd always done 'exceptional things' at the weekend, however, now he's wavering between accepting modestly what he can do (accompanied by feelings of envy and jealousy that arise) or choosing to isolate and shut himself inside a cocoon.

There is the session where he keeps talking about the dialectic between controlling and exploring things, between enclosed and open spaces, and internal and external experience.

At times he sounds nostalgic for the little box where he was enclosed and at other times he expresses his fascination for wide open, unexplored places.

We can see that after six months of work he has begun to shape a rhythm of his own, with a singular intensity of focusing. This is very encouraging.

RP: Luca continues: 'The other day I chaired the Rifondazione meeting. I didn't manage to note it all down, only half. This morning at 7 I went back hoping to meet J and finish the rest with him. I realise from how I chaired the meeting that I don't have the political skill, I'm no leader although I wasn't afraid to talk in public. I cut a rather satisfactory figure even if I was no J.

In class the teachers asked me (I'm the class representative) about whatever has to do with school, and ask U (the classmate who asked to join the school council) about the demonstration in town. This irritated me slightly but U makes the impression of being mature and knowledgeable: people's opinion of him has risen, mine has fallen. I'm little overshadowed by him; once it was me who had the upper hand. With my friend J too there's some conflict: I work much harder for the school paper but students take their poems to him. Sometimes I feel useless and left aside. I used to consider U a notch below me – this irritates me and this is why I tend to keep to myself. When in contact with others I've noticed I've lagged behind – others no longer turn to me, others have surpassed me, I'm no longer the centre of attention; I want to stay at home with a book, isolate myself, closed up in my shelter, and let things go. I no longer torment myself because of these questions. If girls look at U – so be it. Quit all these ideas of how to perform in bed and read Henry Miller. 'Womb and shells … in the hollow of the womb I'm collecting buttercups' (he quotes). 'The womb is big, man is small. It's difficult not to feel envious or jealous of certain things … J's got a creative mind. I'm afraid of disappointing others. I'd like to conserve this and that: the first thing I notice is the awkwardness, inadequacy of some of my ways of behaving.'

DM: Here it becomes clear why and which ambitions emerge: competition within a group, being the centre of attention in a group, amongst male members who seek admiration and do everything to please girls; this is the fundamental ethos in a group of boys at this age.

The rhythm of latency corresponds to the rhythm of the parents: the work week is followed by Saturday night when the father is gratified by a likely sexual encounter with the mother; and on Sunday comes the day of earned rest after accomplishing the weekly duties. This rhythm translates itself into puberty too when a student, after going to school the entire week, expects Saturday night to be his deserved reward, and Sunday is experienced as the day of rest. This rhythm in latency is translated into masturbation and in puberty maybe into an encounter with a prostitute.

But all this is speaking in generalities; here we have a boy with a good nature, a boy who loves his parents and therefore is taken up with the desire to please everyone at the same time. In fact he says he fears disappointing anyone, and as a result he finds himself trapped in falsehoods where he has to practically ask himself: 'But is there a way, what is the system for satisfying everyone at the same time?' He can adopt quite a puritan attitude on the one hand, and can also play a political leader, and generally seems to have found a way to satisfy everyone a little, which is the very essence of this 'system' which he feels he needs to explain and analyse.

RP: The last session is about the school occupation.

Last recent session

Luca begins: 'There are loads of things to tell you; I haven't slept for two nights. My relations with others have improved immensely, especially with my school mates – I'm the head watchman: we've set up a group of about 40 people in charge of controlling all the gates and doors at school. I'm one of those in charge; I have to set up the shifts and make sure they are put into practice; it's a wonderful experience. There are about 800 students at my school, of these 350 to 400 have joined the occupation of the school. In the afternoon we're 150 to 200, the number goes down to 40 at night. It's a test of strength with myself. At night the police came: they told us we risked prison sentences from six months to two years, they threatened us. I felt quite confident, because my family supports me. We (J,U and I) make up the 'hard core'; others wanted to leave – but it was important to stay there, be on the spot; the headmaster didn't ask us to clear the school premises. The first night was strange perhaps because it was the first time; no-one restrained their energies. My shift ran from 2 to 4 in the morning; I had to keep watch in the courtyard. Fatigue … dead silence … there were two of us on the shift, there were moments when we experienced something amazing and moments of intimacy. After the shift I tried to sleep but my sleeping bag was gone: no big deal. Wake up at 6; the following day a massive demonstration with roughly 5000 students – the biggest that has ever happened in my town. I was thrilled. I met M for the first time in two weeks. It was wonderful – we spent the night together. At the demonstration I also saw my father; for the first time since I'd been away from home I could stand together with my girlfriend in front of my parents. In the afternoon I went home to sleep for two hours.

DM: Where did they spend the night together?

RP: Most likely at school.

DM: Without even a sleeping bag?

RP: Luca carries on: 'The afternoon shifts went well; my mates who were on shift the night before were exhausted, some were still asleep, they needed new people. The second night, a quiet night, I was on shift with a girl from the first year, in charge of the entrance hall. We also went out together; I had no particular intentions, she was too young, three years younger than me, in fact I tried to keep away from her. I accompanied her and then I got raped: I couldn't bring myself to say no to her. It was like a dream – I had met her in Rome – then I couldn't sleep (she is the sister of a friend of mine) …'.

DM: After he's somehow succeeded in satisfying everyone (the group, his family), after taking up the role of the policeman, now comes the moment when he gets raped and this is the measure of his infidelity. Here again conflicts come up and everything is put at stake. And he has the feeling that what's wrong with him is his temper, as when he says: 'I couldn't bring myself to say no to her' and so he obliged her wishes.

In fact he meant to deny his desire for this girl, which was essentially his fear, the feeling of uncertainty of reaching an erection, being impotent as he had clearly been with M shortly before.

RP: He continues: 'Which is why when you do these things … in the family, I feel constrained. And there is the problem with A' (a former girl friend). 'I felt bad. I slept with a lot of girlfriends without having anything. They took it for something else – it's really worrying now. I'm in charge of the watches. On the train I calmed down' (here he means the train ride to come to the sessions). 'When at home I'm anxious about a likely eviction – everything is tense. At the meeting this morning we decided at least 100 people were needed to continue the occupation. I don't want to quit – it's a real issue. I'm putting myself into this even though I'm lucky to have my parents on my side (unlike others). Someone had to run away from home to join the occupation. My father has become a hero. He supported us and quarrelled with the security forces. This is a truly important experience, even all these small matters – going up and down the arcades, doing the night rounds, the school lift, up and down the upper floors. I walk round, go into classes. I don't care about aesthetics. The first day I put on boots but then changed into sneakers; I haven't combed my hair, nor washed, a feeling of relief. I feel free; I have given up looking after myself (I can't keep polishing my looks). I've even put on the specs again (which I used to feel ashamed of and had stopped wearing).

'Now I'm doing things which come out here and which we often talk about: sometimes I help someone, sometimes I ask for help and feel I can do it. I ask for moral support. Yesterday I asked U for help, needed to have a talk; I couldn't have done so before. I'm right in it personally. I ring this and that person … the one thing I haven't done so far is ask to have a word at the assemblies' (Luca has told me of his fear of speaking before others). 'Some teachers have stopped greeting me. They claim I've swept the entire class behind me – mine is the class with the highest number of students joining the occupation. Apparently I have passed on the inflammation, I'm overheated. I'm happy I'm responsible for something and feel involved in it right up to my neck. The most amazing thing is the great space at our disposal' (here I think of the story of the box where he was enclosed). 'The long corridors, big labs – an immense building at my disposal. I enjoy walking in these deserted corridors, doing the rounds.'

He sounds worried however; says he has had no time to dream; and that just then, in the session, he has a painful cramp in his leg. Then he goes back to talking about the girl with whom he spent the first night: 'I'm afraid of being considered a son of a bitch, it was a mistake, nice but embarrassing. I like her because she's simple and spontaneous, no beating about the bush. This worries me a little should the affair go on – how should I hide my sexual problems … During the train journey here I had a break to think and there's something I'm terrified of, it's the thought of being sent away from school. I'm afraid they'll evict us; when I get there in the evening I'm afraid of it – so there I don't even smoke so as not to be a bad example. I haven't touched a drop of drink …'.

DM: Here we note there is a very quick development towards identification with his parents and particularly his father, who changes from being the black sheep of the family to a sort of hero at the school occupation whose political reasons I don't know. At any rate, Luca considers himself lucky to have support from his family and in one way or another has managed to rehabilitate his own parents, in order to prevent the figure of the mother from persecuting, monopolizing over him, for example concerning his sexual desire. We could reflect here on his dream about the company of an elderly woman, who is the mother, by contrast with the thirteen-year-old with whom he's had an affair. The boy has got into a position where he thinks that, in order to overcome his difficulties and find an answer to his problems, he should become so attractive as not to need to play an active role any longer but instead can be passive and leave it to the girls to take the initiative and shoulder responsibility. But at this point he gets upset and says: 'No, that's not right, it's not responsible, it's not an honourable objective' – which is why he feels there's something wrong with him.

It's clear he is extremely drawn towards political engagement which for him basically means speaking. Speaking is an important factor for him, and the better he can speak in public the worthier he'll be of admiration and respect. The problem of speaking in public means a lot to him and he feels he needs to get over his fear of it.

This could perhaps provide us with a reason for saying that, as in this case, it's not always and only the bad boys who attack their parents in an attempt to kill them, but also good boys, and some even do it from good motives.

What began with the kindness and thoughtfulness shown by not wishing to commit suicide so as not to make his parents suffer is then transferred to a situation where the boy wishes to avoid forcing his own sexual desire on a girl, precisely in order to prevent her from being disappointed in his sexual performance: in other words, this is a case of distortion of what is in essence a boy with a gentle heart.

CHAPTER ELEVEN

On negative transference
(2001)[1]

Donald Meltzer

I have been asked to give a short talk on negative transference. First of all I'd begin by debunking the notion of negative transference in the sense of hostility, absence of trust, etc. This is a completely mistaken concept when referred to and used in this way. We need to start with Bion's method of classification: the emotional links L, H and K: (love, hate, knowledge) and minus L, minus H, minus K. Let's then look into the negative aspects of love, hate and knowledge: –L, –H, –K. It is these elements that describe the emotional attitude and orientation.

Clearly, to have an idea of positivity, we first need to have an idea of negativity, otherwise it makes no sense. For instance, what does –L, minus love, correspond to? It corresponds to puritanism. By –H, minus hate, we mean hypocrisy. By –K, minus knowledge, we mean philistinism. So these are transference attitudes, each resulting in a countertransference consequence.

Let's first look at the countertransference that occurs with puritanism, in –L. It's a negative link which could be called

---

1   A talk given at a conference organised by the Racker Group; translated.

a confusion, a type of not-understanding, in short the very absence of countertransference. So the transference attitude is felt in the countertransference as incomprehension: experienced by the therapist in terms of a complacent attitude towards the patient.

The negative link of H, that is –H, is the patient's denial of any feelings of hate. I'd call it hypocrisy, which is also linked with a countertransference of incomprehension; this countertransference reveals itself in an attitude of pomposity towards the patient: an attitude of criticising from top to bottom. To sum up, we see that the negative link of L (–L) takes the form of an attitude of incomprehension and complacency in the countertransference; while the negative link of H (–H) results also in incomprehension and in a critical, pompous attitude.

As for –K, philistinism, here also we can observe incomprehension, an inability to think and understand. The patient feels the analyst regards him as stupid. Well, all these types of countertransference experience cause confusion in the therapist, who no longer knows what mode of talking to employ in communicating with the patient, who on his side uses language filled with violence and aggression. The therapist's interpretations are perceived by the patient as given in a negative manner, hence as filled with judgement, pomposity, or the intention of making him feel stupid.

The technical question then of how to convey the existence of this –K element as though it were merely a factual observation means dealing with truly enormous difficulties in order to overcome the patient's hostility and open up a genuine dialogue. On the patient's side it's equally difficult to overcome such an attitude, as he perceives the therapist's words as offensive, aggressive, and intended solely to attack and criticise him; this explains the difficulty of the impasse.

Now, all these negative relations and the resulting countertransference have one thing in common: lack of imagination and fantasy. The patient's inability is one of failing to understand the nature of positive relations, the true significance behind words like love, hate, knowledge; he is unable to understand their true meaning; to him they are just words without significance; he doesn't know what it means to love, hate, or be interested in others.

What then are the consequences? We note that a common element – boredom – ensues when the analyst perceives the patient's inability to imagine, his inability to understand. The boredom is felt both by the therapist towards the patient, and the patient towards the therapist. This boredom can be heard in the nature, the timbre of the patient's voice. Once again if the therapist seeks to describe this feature of the patient's voice, he'll perceive this as an outright assault, an attack. But as it is the patient himself who ultimately is the one who describes his boredom, his own words can be pinpointed in order to analyse the concept of boredom. What lies behind, or underneath this boredom? Once the elements – the things the patient describes which result in boredom – can be analysed, then the analyst can interpret them as absence of interest; it is the absence of interest that causes boredom.

At this stage one could try and show the patient that what he fails to find interesting is the functioning of his own mind. This may stimulate him to the discovery that in his own head a hidden function may in fact make him do interesting things. For instance in Sarah's case, you can see that the patient herself discovers that in her head there is some interesting function which makes her good at designing things. So starting from this area which does seem to engage her interest, it could be useful to go down deeper to see what she finds so interesting in her drawings and in her talent for design.

From a merely technical point of view, the problem the analyst encounters is that he must simply wait for the patient to state or describe a certain situation of element as boring; the patient should be the one to open the discourse on boredom, which in most cases does not take long. Boredom is a universal feeling we are all familiar with; it crops up at the age of six or seven on reaching school age, when a child starts to discover that there may be other children who know how to do things that he doesn't. In this context Sarah discovers her ability to draw and begins making drawings some people find interesting, while others find them uninteresting or boring. What is astonishing is that she herself cannot make out, cannot understand whether her drawings are interesting or boring. Therefore the method consists in opening up that area in the negative grid and observing what is happening and what is not happening. Any page in her case presentation would be enough to illustrate this act of negativity in process. For example the passage where Sarah says: 'Oh yes, I hardly go out, I stay at home with my mother, go out with my friends very rarely', and the therapist says: 'At this stage I almost wish she would break up with Federico, like a parent with an adolescent child who keeps worrying her and who tends to think: well once she leaves her bad friends all her problems will automatically disappear.' The therapist adds: 'But in actual fact, in her relation with Federico the patient might be pouring out all the drugged parts of herself' or something similar. In this case we note the countertransference taking place in the patient's negative link of minus –H. And here we all acknowledge, as does she, that she is being dragged into and getting entangled in a rather stupid relationship. Here we can trace all the elements mentioned earlier: puritanism, as when we make a negative assessment of her sexual choice because she keeps up her relationship with Federico; arrogance and pomposity, as when she pronounces judgement on aspects of her drug addiction and the money Federico should pay her back. Similarly, we can step out from Sarah's experience of drug addiction, using it as a cue to stimulate her to talk about her emotional experience when taking drugs, and her need for comfort.

So, generally speaking, this is the way to open up the negative grid of –L, –H and –K so that you can convey these concepts to the patient in words, although at first it may have an offensive ring, as though the patient were coming under attack. Then move on to the observation of phenomena in which the patient's interest seems to lodge. In a similar fashion, taking the example of Sarah's case, look more closely into the significance of her dependence on social relations, be it her friends or acquaintances, which could be described as if it too were a drug addiction. Look at what happens when she leaves home to live elsewhere, when in fact she does nothing but busy herself with the daily routine of sleeping, eating, dressing and washing etc – till a stage is reached at which these transactions of everyday life are carried out no longer at home but outside home, after which these functions cease altogether so that she stops sleeping, eating, washing herself to the point of stinking. Perhaps, sooner or later, however reluctantly, she'll admit not smelling good, especially on a hot day, well – the nose tells the story!

This brings us back to the core feature of the psychoanalytical work, which is founded on pure and simple observation, neither information nor hearsay; we need to limit ourselves to observing how the patient is dressed, the smell he emanates, if from one session to the next he is getting weaker or thinner, etc. This is the entire basis of analysis, whose material as I have said must be based on observation. The moment one adheres strictly to observation and points out to the patient what is being observed, one needs to be ready to accept and to appreciate some very strong, aggressive and bitter complaints, too.

This is why the negative transference needs to be explored, or rather –L, –H, –K, because analysis is a very interesting process which makes one look into the use and importance of speech, of the possibility of lying, of the exploitation of truth, perhaps by taking a piece of truth and turning it into a lie. All this is highly fruitful psychoanalytical work and at the same time anything but boring.

Sarah's material, on the other hand, I did find boring at points, and she herself is aware of it; she thinks she is bored because she is caught up in some repetitive, boring vicious circle, and expresses her boredom and perplexity. But once this sort of work starts unfolding, the process becomes extremely interesting and lively even though the patient may become aggressive, hostile, and use unpleasant language, even accompanied by threats of suicide or of abandoning the therapy altogether.

From a theoretical point of view it's very useful to analyse this negative grid, although it is difficult to define what the negative grid is. If we have to define it we can do it by antithesis: by stating what is the opposite of thinking, describing the grid for not thinking. When we start to do so we make interesting discoveries, even in this inability to think or imagine on the part of the patient. It's as if there were a voice inside their minds telling them what to say, a little as though they were talking under the influence of narcotics, in a state of hallucination.

I believe it's very useful for the therapist. This is a situation where you can learn a great deal from the patient when they get unpleasant, start being presumptuous, a know-all, and critical of the therapist: 'Ah well, yes but I remember once a year ago, a month ago, you told me …' and so on. This can be very informative. You get to a stage of continuous quarrelling; the consulting room transforms into a battlefield; session after session it's as if an ongoing confrontation were taking place. It's similar to being in a courtroom with lawyers on both sides attacking one another, each uttering only half-truths. Such a process can certainly be highly instructive, albeit equally tiresome. The point is how do you manage to assess if the patient is actually making any progress, when he himself states exactly the opposite, as when he threatens to do terrible things, kill himself, abandon analysis?

I think gauging any likely progress on the patient's side entails an equally simply method of evaluation: it consists in analysing the level, as it were, of the 'noise' produced by the patient. This means facing a truly difficult conflict situation. Obviously, it's hard to keep silent before quite a violent situation, rather than counter-attacking or defending oneself before the patient's provocations and accusations. Of course, you may not succeed, but what you can certainly do is to let the patient exhaust his complaints and energies. What should you do when you're under attack and accused by your patient? It's impossible to defend yourself from the accusations of a patient who states: 'But why, you first said this and now you're saying that, you're contradicting yourself!' It's naturally impossible to remember what you said a month ago, a year ago, etc. The only thing you can say is that the patient is remembering on the basis of paraphrase, and hence what comes out of his mouth is not what was actually said but what he has himself paraphrased. This is how slowly and gradually the noise, the ruminating, of the patient tends to diminish. While this noise dies down, the tone of his voice tends to alter, too; consequently you will no longer note in his voice the aggressive or harsh, accusatory note of fooling and ridiculing what we have said. Nor will you hear the sharp reproach and contempt directed at the therapist's words; the atmosphere will change and the severe, negative tones will give way to softer ones which are not necessarily the speech of love-making but certainly could be defined as gentleness, the opposite of attack.

As the voice changes its tone, becoming ever softer, you may notice a different bodily attitude, changes in posture both in facial movement and in and the body language of the patient. So, this is how the positive transference slowly begins to appear, even if it may take years to do so: years which can prove difficult but no doubt also very interesting.

CHAPTER TWELVE

Current considerations on autism
(2002)[1]

Donald Meltzer

T wenty years ago, I happened to write with a group a book called *Explorations in Autism*. It was such a bad experience that I vowed never to repeat it. I must acknowledge I'm not good at organising groups, and on that occasion rather than a proper group this was a set of highly independent persons; I found myself in the role of a slave master to keep them all together; eventually I wrote the entire book by myself, which is why I vowed I'd never undertake the experience of writing a book with a group again.

An important thing that emerged is that in actual fact autism is very difficult to define, consisting of a lot of disparate points that need to be brought together. In fact, not only do autistic children differ extremely from one another, but the psychoanalytical process that is established also varies from case to case. What we did during those months of work was to take into consideration the different variety of material we had at our disposal, to try to come to a definition of a pure concept of autism. Some of

---

1   A talk given at a conference on autism organised by the Racker Group; translated.

the notions created then have proved their validity in time, they have survived, while others have been replaced.

I notice that what changed most has been the attitude, the approach towards autism. One of those surviving notions concerns dismantling of objects. The notion of dismantling of objects does not refer only to objects but also to the experience of time and space. What gradually grew clearer in the course of this work was that autism is a style, a way of life. The focal point of this new way of understanding autism as a way of life is the notion of 'the *idiot savant* disorder'. The phenomenon of *idiot savant* constitutes the principle characteristic of autism. There are more than a few *idiot savants* full of gift and talent, not just in the field of painting but also of music. The diffusion of this phenomenon, that is of autistic people particularly gifted in artistic fields, has meant considering the autistic phenomena at present in terms of a different mentality from those we have generally known and accepted. In addition, what has in my view emerged very particularly is a different attitude towards an autistic person's success or not in integrating himself.

As the process of growth gradually unfolds, the process of symbol formation also develops. Just this morning I read an article by Ellie Roberts who has an autistic child of nine in therapy who is making enormous progress in his development. This child is also seeing an artist who is employing artistic methods for the therapy. At the beginning the child had urinary and faecal incontinence, was hyperactive and could not speak; little by little he has made enormous progress in all these areas, perhaps thanks to the relationship with the art therapist even more than the psychotherapist. This child's mother is a very strict woman, wooden in demeanour, with absolutely no imagination, and extremely literal-minded; she can observe facts but is unable to go beyond them to get to their significance; yet she is also very patient with her child. The parents of this child have separated; he is the youngest of their three children and the only one with serious developmental problems. As I mentioned, the child's relation with the art therapist, a joyful, dynamic and very engaging man, has proved particularly strong. The child turned out to be attracted by colours, painting, coloured paper, brushes and so on as tools of representation.

Question: Had the art therapist employed another technique, would the result be the same? Does the technique have any effect or is it the person who has managed to establish a good relation? Is it the person or the technique that establishes the transference relation?

Donald Meltzer: Who knows! This is a difficult question to answer; the answer might come out gradually from the material of analysis. Indeed, this child seemed to enjoy handling the materials: he would press and squeeze the paint tubes, play with the brushes and use them to colour paintings. His mother showed a lot of resistance to this therapy technique and at one point wanted to take him away; but the art therapist insisted she should let the cihld try again and succeeded in convincing her to stay to see how things would prove. As she was a very concrete person, she didn't want him to squeeze out all those paint tubes, thinking the paint was being wasted. The art therapist had to convince her that she need not worry as there were a lot of paint tubes and the child did not squeeze out the paint completely. The mother calmed down and this is how they carried on with the work. In one of the sessions the child was given a green sheet of paper and he decided to paint black upon it. The two therapists who were looking on were surprised to see the result: an elliptical drawing the child said was like a face and which had the clear shape of a mouth, nose, eyes and eyebrows. Then he drew another thing he said was like a hand; afterwards he put the brush in his mouth and started sucking it; in a moment of distraction the art therapist told him he mustn't put the brush in his mouth and the child was very hurt as he felt he was being limited in his expressiveness and turned his back to the art therapist. His mother, who was there too, noticed the child's reaction and intervened, trying to comfort him; she told her son the art therapist had done so to protect him, not to punish him. On hearing these words the child took up the brush again, soaked it in black and started painting his mother's face below the eyes. His mother, strangely enough, made no move to stop him and despite her discomfort let him paint her face. Soon he grew bored with this and stopped painting; he then went up to the toolbox, took out a crocodile, and held it towards his mother as though it meant to eat her up while saying 'I'm hungry'. He then almost lay down by his mother, leaning towards her breast as if he meant to suck at it; he turned the crocodile round with the tail directed towards her breast; again, surprisingly, his mother seemed to tolerate the game with the crocodile, its teeth and tail; it was as if the child caressed her with the crocodile's tail while she reacted warmly, welcoming him.

I interpret this material on a part-object level: the crocodile with its sharp teeth as if it were the father's penis, besides being that of the art therapist who had told off the child. Thanks to the warm and indulgent reaction of the mother, who had accepted her son's play not as something aggressive but as an attempt to caress her with the tail of the crocodile, I read this as a good answer from the child's side to try to put together, reassemble, reunify the combined object of the penis–breast. At this point the mother took out a tissue to wipe the paint off her face.

I don't see the child's gesture as intended to disfigure his mother's face; on the contrary, it seems intended to make it friendlier, warmer. I also read the hand he drew earlier as a split object: the father's penis that admonishes him for sucking at his mother's breast. The scene we were witnessing, in my view, was a glimpse of the autistic mentality which focused on not just the splitting of objects but also on their reunification, their reassembly. Moreover, it suggests something far more sophisticated – the child's attempt to forgive his mother. How? By transforming her frowning face into one with a smile on it. Another thing we noticed was that at the end as the child was going out, he put his hand on the art therapist's knee as a gesture of forgiveness, just as he had forgiven his mother earlier.

All this could seem a highly exaggerated interpretation of some very minimal activity; but no matter how minimal it may be, it's amazing that such an autistic child had expressed so much through these minimal actions, that is by painting a face, by representing a hand as something distinct from a face, and by using his mother's face as a sheet of paper to paint with a brush full of meaning; moreover, he had been able to say in his own way 'I forgive you even if you behaved badly'; he showed he'd accepted his mother's pardon and that he could reconstruct this warmth.

Why did I describe this scene in such detail to you? Why did I speak about it? Just to emphasise the need for careful and meticulous observation, imaginative and creative observation. It seems clear the therapist not only acted in a way that meant the mother would not interrupt the therapy but also helped her to get interested in the process itself; he had her brought in. It's important to note how the two therapists worked together to succeed in engaging and interesting the mother so that she too could take part in what was happening to her child in the course of the therapy.

What is meant by creative imagination? This is what Wittgenstein called 'seeing-as', which is the opposite of concreteness; it's observing the inner sense of things. In the case we are considering, imaginative creativity has been the turning point in the development of the therapy: the ability to imagine that the child was employing painting to draw a new face for his mother, bringing her into the process of therapy, inducing a change in his mother's attitude, arousing her interest and making her accept, with fun and humour as well, even to get stained. There's much to be learned from imaginative capacity. Nothing is as it looks! The sense always lies hidden.

I am thinking of Velasquez' use of mirrors within a painting; the sense of his activity is represented in that mirror. In *The Rokeby Venus*, this is seen in the reflection in the mirror Cupid holds, whose angle shows that Venus is looking not at her own reflection but at that of the artist. In *Las Meninas* there is a mirror, too; the artist depicts himself while looking at the scene through an open door, as though from a different perspective; this is a formidable way to represent Wittgenstein's notion of 'seeing-as'. Bion names such imaginative changes of perspective 'vertices'. In children's games we see this when they take out sand from the toolbox, form small heaps, stick little trees into them and then lie down to look at the landscape as though it were perhaps a beach. While observing their behaviour, we need to consider 'seeing-as', that is, to observe imaginatively in order to see not just what is on the surface but to be able to reach the meaning of their behaviour. To understand the meaning we must shift our vertex.

I am particularly fond of the painting *Las Meninas* because the artist actually has two perspectives: the first where he is seen in the foreground while painting the group, the second when he himself is part of the painted scene, reflected in a mirror.

The rule of observing imaginatively seems particularly important, it offers a different viewpoint on life, sometimes a highly complex and interesting one. I find one of the most impressive windows on imaginative thinking in Bion's formulation of alpha-function and his idea that alpha elements can be cannibalised by a reversal of this function and converted into bizarre objects with traces of ego and superego.

The two vertices on autism which I consistently adopt after 20 years of working with and taking an interest in autistic children are the following: firstly, autism is a variant of thinking and development which is based on the reversal of alpha-function; and secondly, it involves projective identification on a part-object level. By applying imaginatively these two principles the autistic material can be interpreted in the same way as interpreting dreams. I know this may sound trifling after all those years of work but believe me, this represents the key to understanding the phenomenon of the *idiot savant* and the way his mind works; it makes us understand that we are not dealing with mental disorder but with a special form of thinking and development. Besides, in my view the *idiot savants* are, far more frequently than we suppose, among the geniuses of the world, the gifted and talented people.

The case we discussed this morning in supervision is not an *idiot savant* case,[2] nor is it the case of an autistic patient, but we can define the case in terms of 'a patient with autistic features'. If we examine meticulously the way her hallucinations work like a satanic voice, we may see that those hallucinations function just like the reversal of alpha-function. In Bion's quite prophetic words: to be able to lie you first need to know the truth. In

---

2   See Chapter 4.

this patient we saw today and in her dream-life we can observe how the truth is being warped by this hallucinatory satanic voice which distorts the truth into a lie. The danger of this lie is represented in the dream about 'anthrax pie'; this describes in a concrete way the effect of the lie on people's minds, because it can become almost a truth, and therefore have a truly negative influence on life itself. Lies are the poison of the mind.